W0035870

Small Animal
DRUG HANDBOOK

Small Animal
DRUG HANDBOOK

RHEA V. MORGAN, DVM
Diplomate
American College of Veterinary Internal Medicine and
  American College of Veterinary Ophthalmologists
Smoky Mountain Veterinary Services
Walland, Tennessee

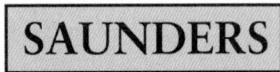
An Imprint of Elsevier Science

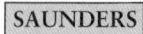

An Imprint of Elsevier Science

11830 Westline Industrial Drive
St. Louis, Missouri 63146

NOTICE

Veterinary Medicine is an ever-changing field. Standard safety precautions
must be followed, but as new research and clinical experience broaden
our knowledge, changes in treatment and drug therapy may become
necessary or appropriate. Readers are advised to check the most current
product information provided by the manufacturer of each drug to be
administered to verify the recommended dose, the method and dura-
tion of administration, and contraindications. It is the responsibility of
the licensed prescriber, relying on experience and knowledge of the
patient, to determine dosages and the best treatment for each individual patient. Neither the publisher nor the author assumes any liability
for any injury and/or damage to persons or property arising from this
publication.

International Standard Book Number 0-7216-0124-3

Acquisitions Editor: Ray Kersey
Developmental Editor: Denise LeMelledo
Project Manager: Joy Moore
Designer: Julia Dummitt

Printed in United States of America

Last digit is the print number: 9   8   7   6   5   4   3   2   1

Preface

Welcome to the *Small Animal Drug Handbook*. This formulary has been compiled from the 4th Edition of the *Handbook of Small Animal Practice (HSAP)*, which was published in September 2002. The material presented here represents just a small portion of the extensive body of work prepared for this latest edition of the *HSAP*.

This booklet is composed of four different sections. Section I provides lists of the common units used for weights, fluids, and pressures, and the commonly used abbreviations for routes of administration and dosage schedules. It also contains descriptions of the abbreviations used within the formulary. Section II is the actual drug formulary. Drugs are listed in alphabetical order by generic name. Under each drug, one or more uses of the drug are listed, and these are followed by the dosages recommended for that particular condition. The chapter number(s) from the *HSAP* where the drug is cited are also provided so that the text pertaining to the drug and disease process can readily be reviewed. At the beginning of Section II there is a key that explains the format of the entries and prefixes used in the formulary. Section III is an alphabetical list of the drugs by brand name. Section IV provides a classification of the drugs by their type or activity, and the drugs are listed by generic name.

Section II of this drug handbook corresponds to Appendix IV of the 4th Edition of the *HSAP*. To make this material more mobile and usable in clinical practice, not only have we created this small pocket-sized booklet, but we are also making the material available in an electronic format for use on a personal digital assistant (PDA). The PDA CD-ROM can be obtained from bookstores and retail outlets, as well as from Elsevier Health Sciences' website at www.elsevierhealth.com. The PDA version can also be downloaded from the website. The PDA version of this booklet is compatible with PalmOS, Windows CE, and Pocket PC devices.

We hope that this format of presenting drugs by specific usage and dosage regimen will provide clinical veterinarians with a precise, accurate, and practical tool — one that will prove highly useful on a daily basis.

Rhea V. Morgan DVM
Diplomate ACVIM, ACVO
Senior Editor, *Handbook of Small Animal Practice*
October 2002

Contents

Small Animal
DRUG HANDBOOK

Units, Abbreviations, Equivalents

Units

Weights

oz	ounce
lb	pound
kg	kilograms (10^3 g)
g	gram (1 g)
mg	milligram (10^{-3} g)
μg	microgram (10^{-6} g)
ng	nanogram (10^{-9} g)
pg	picogram (10^{-12} g)
gr	grain (1 gr = 65 mg)

Fluids

L	liter (10^3 ml)
dl	deciliter (10^2 ml)
ml	milliliter (1 ml or 10^{-3} L)
μl	microliter (10^{-6} L)
tsp	teaspoon
tbsp	tablespoon

Pressure

mmHg	millimeters of mercury
cm H_2O	centimeters of water

Distance, Surface Area

mm	millimeters
cm	centimeters
in.	inches
m^2	meter squared

Time

sec	second
min	minute
hr, h	hour
q	every

day	day
wk	week
mo	month
yr	year

Concentration of Solutions

mEq/L	milliequivalents per liter
g/dl	grams per deciliter
mg/dl	milligrams per deciliter
pg/dl	picograms per deciliter
mOsm/kg	milliosmoles per kilogram
μU/ml	microunits per milliliter
μg/dl	micrograms per deciliter
μmol/L	micromoles per liter
mmol/L	millimoles per liter
pmol/L	picomoles per liter
mmol/kg	millimoles per kilogram
g/L	grams per liter
U/L	units per liter
IU/L	international units per liter
ppm	parts per million

Modified from Morgan RV: Manual of Small Animal Emergencies. Churchill Livingstone, New York, 1985.

Abbreviations

Routes of Administration

PO	per os, oral
IC	intracardiac
IM	intramuscular
IV	intravenous
SC	subcutaneous
IT	intrathecal
IO	intraosseous
IP	intraperitoneal

Dosage Schedules

QID	four times daily; every 6 hours
TID	three times daily; every 8 hours
BID	twice daily; every 12 hours
SID	once daily; every 24 hours
QOD	once every other day; every 48 hours
q	every

Other Abbreviations Used in the Formulary

ADH	Antidiuretic hormone
AV	Atrioventricular
BUN	Blood urea nitrogen
CNS	Central nervous system
CPR	Cardiopulmonary resuscitation
CRI	Continuous rate infusion
dd	Divided dose
DIC	Disseminated intravascular coagulation
DJD	Degenerative joint disease
D/W	Dextrose in water
EPI	Exocrine pancreatic insufficiency
FeLV	Feline leukemia virus
FIP	Feline infectious peritonitis
FIV	Feline immunodeficiency virus
FSH	Follicle-stimulating hormone
FUS	Feline urologic syndrome
GI	Gastrointestinal
IO	Intraosseously
IT	Intrathecally
KCS	Keratoconjunctivitis sicca
max	Maximum
NSAID	Nonsteroidal anti-inflammatory drug
PCV	Packed cell volume
PRN	As needed
Rx	Treatment
SA	Sinoatrial
SLE	Systemic lupus erythematosus
soln	Solution
tab	Tablet
URI	Upper respiratory infection

Equivalents of Centigrade (Celsius) and Fahrenheit Temperatures

°C	°F
23	73.4
24	75.2
25	77.0
26	78.8
27	80.6
28	82.4
29	84.2
30	86.0
31	87.8
32	89.6
33	91.4
34	93.2
35	95.0
36	96.8
37	98.6
38	100.4
39	102.2
40	104.0
41	105.8
42	107.6
43	109.4
44	111.2
45	113.0
46	114.8

Formulary

Every effort has been made to provide precise dosages for specific clinical situations; however, individual needs or circumstances may necessitate alterations in both the dosage and the frequency of administration of any of the medications listed on the following pages. Dosages are designated for either "Dog" or "Cat." If neither designation appears, the dosage is applicable to both the dog and cat. *Note:* Multiple uses for the drug are listed in order under original drug entry.

Key: **Drug (Brand Name or abbreviation)**
     Purpose or Use
       Chapters cited
       Dosage
       Prefix indicates species
       No prefix indicates dosage is applicable to both
         dog and cat.

Note: Multiple uses for drug are listed in order under original drug entry.

ABBREVIATIONS USED IN THE FORMULARY

ADH	Antidiuretic hormone
AV	Atrioventricular
BUN	Blood urea nitrogen
CNS	Central nervous system
CPR	Cardiopulmonary resuscitation
CRI	Continuous rate infusion
dd	Divided dose
DIC	Disseminated intravascular coagulation
DJD	Degenerative joint disease
D/W	Dextrose in water
EPI	Exocrine pancreatic insufficiency
FeLV	Feline leukemia virus

FIP	Feline infectious peritonitis
FIV	Feline immunodeficiency virus
FSH	Follicle-stimulating hormone
FUS	Feline urologic syndrome
GI	Gastrointestinal
IO	Intraosseously
IT	Intrathecally
KCS	Keratoconjunctivitis sicca
max	Maximum
NSAID	Nonsteroidal anti-inflammatory drug
PCV	Packed cell volume
PRN	As needed
Rx	Treatment
SA	Sinoatrial
SLE	Systemic lupus erythematosus
soln	Solution
tab	Tablet
URI	Upper respiratory infection

■ Acarbose (Precose)
Diabetes mellitus
Chapter 43
DOG: <25 kg: 25–50 mg PO BID
>25 kg: 25–100 mg PO BID
Use with insulin

■ Acetazolamide (Diamox)
Hydrocephalus, neurogenic pruritus
Chapters 23, 82
DOG: 0.1 mg/kg PO TID
Glaucoma
Chapter 98
DOG: 5–10 mg/kg IV × 1–2 doses

■ Acetohydroxamic acid (Lithostat)
Struvite urolithiasis
Chapter 49
DOG: 12.5 mg/kg PO BID

Acetylcysteine (Mucomyst)
Degenerative myelopathy
Chapter 24
DOG: 70 mg/kg PO TID × 2 wk, then TID on alternating
days
Acetaminophen toxicosis
Chapters 63, 122, 128
CAT: 140–240 mg/kg PO or 140 mg/kg IV, then 70 mg/kg
PO QID × 5–7 Rx

Acetylpromazine (Acepromazine)
Restraint, sedation
Chapters 4, 15, 37, 59, 79
DOG: 0.025–0.2 mg/kg IV; max = 2.5 mg or
0.1–0.25 mg/kg IM/SC/PO
CAT: 0.025–0.1 mg/kg IV; max = 1 mg
Arterial thromboembolism
Chapter 10
0.1–0.2 mg/kg SC TID
Scotty cramps
Chapter 23
DOG: 0.1–0.75 mg/kg PO BID
Preanesthetic
Chapter 32
DOG: 0.1–0.2 mg/kg IV/IM; max = 2.5 mg
Vertigo
Chapter 106
DOG: 1 mg/kg PO SID
Amphetamine toxicosis
Chapters 122, 128
0.05–1 mg/kg IV/IM/SC, with caution

Acetylsalicylic acid (Aspirin)
Antithrombic, antiprostaglandin effects
Chapters 10, 18
DOG: 10 mg/kg PO BID
CAT: 6–15 mg/kg PO q 48–72 h

Acetylsalicylic acid (Aspirin) *(continued)*
Glomerulonephritis
Chapter 47
DOG: 0.5 mg/kg PO SID–BID
Musculoskeletal pain, inflammation
Chapters 24, 78, 79
DOG: 10–25 mg/kg PO BID–TID
CAT: 6 mg/kg PO q 48–72 h
Antipyretic, analgesic, ocular effects
Chapters 70, 71, 84, 96, 97, 101
DOG: 5–10 mg/kg PO SID–BID
CAT: 3–6 mg/kg PO q 48–72 h

Acitretin (Soriatane)
Keratinization defects, sebaceous adenitis,
keratoacanthoma
Chapters 82, 85, 88, 91
DOG: 0.5–1 mg/kg PO SID

Aclarubicin
Myelodysplastic syndrome
Chapter 65
DOG: 5 mg/m^2 IV SID × 5 days

Actinomycin D (Cosmegen)
Chemotherapy
Chapter 70
DOG: 0.5–0.9 mg/m^2 IV slowly q 3 wk

Activated charcoal (Actidose-Aqua, Requa)
Gastrointestinal adsorbent
Chapters 122–130
1–2 g/5 ml water: give 10 ml of slurry/kg PO

Aglepristone (Alizine) (not available in USA)
Mammary fibroadenomatous hyperplasia
Chapter 59
10 mg/kg SC SID × 4–5 days

Albendazole
Paragonimus, **capillariasis, giardiasis**
    Chapters 18, 47, 114
    25–50 mg/kg PO BID × 7–14 days

Albuterol (Ventolin, Proventil)
Bronchodilator
    Chapters 16, 17, 132
    DOG: 0.02–0.05 mg/kg PO BID–TID

Allopurinol (Zyloprim)
Urate urolithiasis
    Chapters 47, 49
    DOG: 10–15 mg/kg PO BID × 30 days, then 5–7 mg/kg
        PO SID
Leishmaniasis
    Chapters 84, 114
    DOG: 15 mg/kg PO BID, with meglumine antimonate

Alprazolam (Xanax)
FUS
    Chapter 49
    CAT: 0.1–0.2 mg PO SID–BID
Certain behavioral disorders
    Chapters 116, 117
    DOG: 0.01–1.0 mg PO PRN; max = 4 mg/day
    CAT: 2.5–5.0 mg PO SID–BID

Altrenagest (Regumate)
Hypoluteoidism
    Chapter 60
    DOG: 0.088 mg/kg PO SID

Aluminum hydroxide (ALternaGEL, Amphojel)
Phosphate binder
    Chapters 47, 79, 123
    10–30 mg/kg PO BID–TID with meals

Amikacin (Amikin, Amiglyde-V)
Serious infections, endocarditis, osteomyelitis, sepsis
Chapters 9, 31, 79, 110
DOG: 5–15 mg/kg IM/IV/SC SID–TID or 20–30 mg/kg
IV SID
CAT: 10 mg/kg IM/SC/IV TID
Gastroenteritis
Chapter 32
6–8 mg/kg IV SID

Aminocaproic acid (Amicar)
Degenerative myelopathy
Chapter 24
DOG: 500 mg PO TID

Aminophylline (Aminophyllin, Somophyllin)
Bronchodilator
Chapters 9, 17, 18, 132
DOG: 6–11 mg/kg IM/SC/PO TID
CAT: 4–6 mg/kg PO/IM/IV BID

Amitraz (Mitaban)
Demodicosis, sarcoptic mange
Chapter 87
DOG: 5.3 ml/gal water; dip wet dog and air-dry
q 7–14 days × 3–6 Rx

Amitriptyline HCl (Elavil, Amitriptyline)
Certain behavioral disorders, FUS
Chapters 49, 116, 117
DOG: 1–2 mg/kg PO BID
CAT: 2.5–5 mg PO SID–BID
Acral lick granuloma, allergic dermatitis
Chapters 86, 89
DOG: 0.5–2 mg/kg PO BID
CAT: 0.625–1.25 mg PO SID

Amlodipine (Norvasc)
Hypertension, vasodilator
>Chapters 9, 47
>**DOG:** 0.05–0.25 mg/kg PO SID
>**CAT:** 0.625–1.25 mg/cat PO SID

Ammonium chloride (NH$_4$Cl)
Urinary acidifier
>Chapters 122, 123, 128
>**DOG:** 100–200 mg/kg/day PO dd TID–QID
>**CAT:** 20 mg/kg PO BID

Amoxicillin (Amoxidrops, Amoxitabs)
Routine infections
>Chapters 27, 30, 34, 85
>10–20 mg/kg PO/SC/IV BID–TID
>Amoxitabs
Serious infections
>Chapters 33, 51, 60, 84, 101, 111, 112
>20–22 mg/kg PO/SC/IV/IM BID–TID

Amoxicillin/clavulanic acid (Clavamox)
Various bacterial infections
>Chapters 9, 16, 18, 27, 79, 84, 85, 100, 101, 111, 112
>12–22 mg/kg (amoxicillin) PO BID–TID

Amphetamine SO$_4$ (Adderall)
CNS stimulation during certain toxicoses, chlorpromazine overdose
>Chapters 122, 128
>**DOG:** 1–4 mg/kg SC PRN

Amphotericin B (Fungizone)
Systemic mycoses, prototothecosis
>Chapters 14, 32, 100, 109
>**DOG: a)** 0.25–0.50 mg/kg in 0.5–1 L 5% D/W IV over
>6–8 hr; QOD to total dose of 8–10 mg/kg or BUN
>and creatinine levels rise

Amphotericin B (Fungizone) *(continued)*
> **b)** 0.5–0.8 mg/kg diluted in saline and dextrose SC
> 2–3 times weekly (cryptococcosis)
> **CAT:** 0.25 mg/kg IV QOD to total dose of 5–8 mg/kg

Amphotericin, liposomal (Avelcet)
Leishmaniasis, systemic mycoses
> Chapters 32, 100, 109, 114
> **DOG:** 1–3 mg/kg IV QOD to total dose of 12–24 mg/kg

Ampicillin (Omnipen, Polycillin, Polyflex)
Various infections, leptospirosis
> Chapters 9, 24, 27, 31–33, 47, 60, 100–101, 110–112
> 22 mg/kg PO TID or 11–22 mg/kg IV/SC/IM TID–QID

Amprolium (Corid)
Coccidiosis
> **DOG:** 200 mg in food or water PO SID × 7–10 days
> **CAT:** 60–100 mg in food or water PO SID × 5 days

Antidiuretic hormone
> *See* **Desmopressin acetate**

Apomorphine
Induction of vomiting
> Chapter 122
> **DOG:** 0.04 mg/kg IV or 0.08 mg/kg IM/SC or crush small
> amount into conjunctival sac

Ascorbic acid (vitamin C)
Reduction of methemoglobin (acetaminophen toxicity)
> Chapters 122, 124, 128
> 30 mg/kg PO/SC QID × 7 Rx

Ehlers-Danlos syndrome
> Chapter 82
> **DOG:** 500 mg PO BID

Asparaginase (Elspar)
Lymphosarcoma, lymphocytic leukemia, mastocythemia
Chapters 67, 70
DOG: a) 10,000 IU/m^2 IM weekly in a protocol
b) 400 IU/kg IM/SC weekly in a protocol
c) 20,000 IU/m^2 SC in a protocol
CAT: 400 IU/kg IM/SC/IP in a protocol

Atenolol (Tenormin)
Supraventricular tachycardia
Chapters 6, 7, 9, 10, 41
DOG: a) 0.2–1 mg/kg PO SID–BID
b) 6.25–25 mg/dog PO BID
CAT: 6.25–12.5 mg/cat PO SID–BID
Hypertension
Chapter 47
2 mg/kg PO SID–BID

Atipamezole
Amitraz toxicity
Chapter 87
DOG: 0.05 mg/kg IM q 30 min PRN

Atracurium besylate (Tracrium)
Paralytic agent
Chapter 134
DOG: 0.3–0.5 mg/kg IV loading dose, then
4–9 µg/kg/min IV

Atropine SO$_4$
Sinus bradycardia, SA block, AV block
Chapters 7, 8, 74
0.01–0.04 mg/kg IM/SC/IV PRN
Atropine response test
Chapter 7
0.04 mg/kg IM

Atropine SO$_4$ *(continued)*
Preanesthetic
  0.02–0.04 mg/kg SC/IM
Hypersialism
  Chapter 28
  0.02–0.04 mg/kg SC PRN
Cholinergic toxins
  Chapters 122, 124, 129
  0.2–0.5 mg/kg; give one fourth of dose IV, the rest SC/IM

Auranofin (Ridaura)
Autoimmune skin diseases
  Chapter 89
  DOG: 0.1–0.2 mg/kg PO BID

Aurothioglucose (Solganal)
**Plasmacytic stomatitis and pododermatitis,
immune-mediated arthritis**
  Chapters 27, 78, 85
  Test dose of 1–5 mg IM, then 1 mg/kg IM weekly until
    remission, then biweekly or monthly
Pemphigus complex
  Chapter 89
  Test dose of 1 mg IM, then 1 mg IM weekly (<10 kg) or
    5 mg IM weekly (>10 kg)

Azathioprine (Imuran)
Pulmonary eosinophilic diseases
  Chapter 18
  DOG: 2 mg/kg PO SID × 7–10 days, then QOD
Refractory acquired myasthenia gravis
  Chapter 25
  DOG: 2 mg/kg PO SID–QOD
**Lymphocytic/plasmacytic, eosinophilic stomatitis,
gastritis or enteritis**
  Chapters 27, 30, 32
  DOG: 1–2.5 mg/kg PO SID–QOD
  CAT: 0.2–0.3 mg/kg PO SID–QOD
Chronic active hepatitis, glomerulonephritis
  Chapters 34, 47
  DOG: 1–2.5 mg/kg PO SID–QOD

Perianal fistula
 Chapter 36
 DOG: 50 mg PO SID
Immune hemolytic anemia, myelofibrosis
 Chapters 63, 65
 DOG: 2 mg/kg PO SID × 7–10 days, then 1 mg/kg PO
  SID–QOD
Immune thrombocytopenia
 Chapter 66
 DOG: a) 2 mg/kg PO SID, taper to 0.5–1 mg/kg PO QOD
   b) 50 mg/m^2 PO SID, taper to 25 mg/m^2 PO QOD
**Immune skin diseases, SLE, sterile pyogranulomas,
cutaneous histiocytosis**
 Chapters 74, 75, 85, 89, 91
 DOG: 2.2 mg/kg or 50 mg/m^2 PO SID–QOD
Rheumatoid and immune-mediated arthritis
 Chapter 78
 DOG: 2 mg/kg PO SID × 14–21 days, then QOD
**Blepharitis, episcleritis, anterior uveitis, ligneous
conjunctivitis**
 Chapters 93, 94, 96, 97
 DOG: 2 mg/kg PO SID, then taper
**Immune polymyositis, masticatory myositis,
chorioretinitis**
 Chapters 80, 100, 101
 DOG: 2 mg/kg PO SID, eventually taper

Azithromycin (Zithromax)
Campylobacter, Helicobacter, **cryptosporidiosis**
 Chapters 32, 114
 DOG: 5–10 mg/kg PO SID–BID
 CAT: 7–15 mg/kg PO BID × 5–7 days

Baclofen (Lioresal)
Functional urethral obstruction
 Chapter 50
 DOG: 1–2 mg PO TID

BAL
See Dimercaprol

Benazepril (Lotensin)
Hypertension
Chapters 9, 47
DOG: 0.25–0.5 mg/kg PO SID–BID

Benzimidazole
Trypanosomiasis
5 mg/kg PO SID × 2 mo

Betamethasone (Celestone)
Pannus, episcleritis
Chapter 96
DOG: 1–2 mg subconjunctivally

Betaxolol 0.5% (Betoptic)
Selective β-blocker for glaucoma
Chapter 98
Apply 1 drop to affected eye twice daily

Bethanechol (Urecholine)
Bladder atony, dysautonomia
Chapters 50, 103
DOG: 2.5–10.0 mg SC TID or 5–25 mg PO BID–TID
CAT: 1.5–5 mg PO SID–TID

Bisacodyl (Dulcolax)
Stool softener
DOG: 10 mg PO SID PRN
CAT: 5 mg PO SID PRN

Bismuth (Pepto-Bismol)
GI tract protectant, *Helicobacter*
Chapters 30, 32, 33, 111
DOG: 0.25–2 ml/kg PO TID–QID

Bleomycin (Blenoxane)
Chemotherapy
> **DOG:** 10 mg/m^2 IV/SC SID × 4 days, then 10 mg/m^2
> weekly to max dose 200 mg/m^2

Bovine hemoglobin
> *See* Oxyglobin

Bretylium (Bretylium)
Ventricular fibrillation
> Chapter 8
> **DOG:** 5 mg/kg IV; repeat in 5 min

Brinzolamide 1% (Azopt)
Glaucoma
> Chapter 98
> 1 drop to affected eye BID–TID

Bromocriptine (Bromocriptine mesylate)
Galactorrhea
> Chapters 59, 60
> **DOG:** 20–30 μg/kg PO SID × 2–16 days

Buprenorphine (Buprenex)
Analgesia
> Chapters 31, 70, 132
> **DOG:** 0.005–0.15 mg/kg IV/IM/SC TID–QID
> **CAT:** 5–10 μg/kg IM/IV/SC BID–TID or 3–5 μg/kg IV in
> normal saline BID

Buspirone (BuSpar)
Anxiolytic drug
> Chapters 86, 116, 117
> **DOG:** 1–2 mg/kg PO SID
> **CAT:** 5–10 mg/cat PO BID–TID

Busulfan (Myleran)
Chronic granulocytic leukemia
> Chapter 65
> **DOG:** 4 mg/m^2 or 0.1 mg/kg PO SID

Butorphanol tartrate (Torbutrol, Torbugesic)
Cough suppressant
> Chapters 16, 17, 112
> **DOG:** 0.5–1 mg/kg PO BID–QID

Preanesthetic
> 0.05 mg/kg IV or 0.4 mg/kg SC/IM

Analgesia, sedation, restraint
> Chapters 3, 4, 15, 24, 31, 35, 37, 69, 70, 79, 132, 133
> **DOG:** 0.1–0.2 mg/kg IV or 0.2–0.4 mg/kg SC/IM q 2–6 h
> **CAT:** 0.1–0.8 mg/kg IM/SC q 4–6 h

Analgesia
> Chapters 49, 101
> **CAT:** 1 mg PO SID–BID

Cabergoline (Galastop, Dostinex)
Induce estrus
> Chapter 60
> **DOG:** 5 μg/kg PO SID × 7–10 days

Decrease milk production, galactorrhea
> Chapters 59, 60
> **DOG:** 1.5–5.0 μg/kg PO SID × 2–8 days

Calcitonin (Calcimar)
Hypercalcemia, cholecalciferol toxicosis
> Chapters 71, 122, 123
> **DOG:** 4–6 IU/kg SC/IM q 2–12 h

Calcitriol (Rocaltrol)
Hypocalcemia
> Chapter 42
> 5–15 ng/kg PO SID

Chronic renal failure
> Chapters 47, 79
> 1–3 ng/kg PO SID

Seborrhea in cocker spaniels
> Chapter 88
> **DOG:** 10 ng/kg PO SID

■ Calcium carbonate (Caltrate, Tums, Calcet)
Hypocalcemia, eclampsia
> Chapters 42, 60
> 100–150 mg/kg PO dd BID–TID or 1–3 g/day PO

■ Calcium chloride
Ventricular asystole from hyperkalemia
> Chapter 8
> 10% soln: 0.2 ml/kg IV

■ Calcium EDTA (Versenate)
Lead and zinc poisoning
> Chapters 122, 127
> 100 mg/kg/day × 5 days = total dose; make soln of 1 g
> versenate/100 ml 5% D/W, divide total quantity
> milliliters into 20 aliquots, give 1 dose SC QID ×
> 5 days

■ Calcium gluconate (Calcet, Ca gluconate injection)
Ventricular asystole, atrial standstill
> Chapters 7, 8
> 10% soln: 0.4–1.0 ml/kg IV PRN
Hypocalcemia, hyperkalemia
> Chapters 42, 44, 47, 60
> 10% soln:
> a) 0.5–1 ml/kg IV up to 10 ml in 5% D/W over 20–30 min;
>   may repeat at 6- to 8-hr intervals
> b) 20 mg/kg IV infusion in 5% D/W at 22 ml/kg
>   q 8 hr
> Tab: 150–250 mg/kg PO BID–TID
Eclampsia, dystocia
> Chapter 60
> a) 30–100 mg/kg/day PO
> b) 0.2–0.4 ml/kg IM/SC
> c) 1–10 ml IV to effect

Calcium lactate (Calcet, Calphosan)
Hypocalcemia
Chapter 42
130–200 mg/kg PO TID

Captan powder 50% (Orthocide)
Dermatomycoses
Chapter 84
Mix 2 tbsp/gal water, use topically twice weekly; do not rinse after applying

Captopril (Capoten)
Vasodilator, congestive heart failure
Chapter 9
DOG: 0.5–2 mg/kg PO BID–TID

Carboplatin (Paraplatin)
Chemotherapy, in a protocol
Chapters 27, 70, 79
LARGE DOG: 250–300 mg/m^2 IV q 3 wk
SMALL DOG: 10 mg/kg IV q 3 wk
CAT: 150 mg/m^2 IV q 3 wk

Carprofen (Rimadyl)
Analgesia
Chapters 70, 101
DOG: 2 mg/kg PO BID
Musculoskeletal pain or inflammation
Chapters 78, 79
DOG: 2.2 mg/kg PO BID
Anterior uveitis
Chapters 96, 97
DOG: 2 mg/kg PO BID

L-Carnitine (Tyson)
Nutritional supplement, cardiomyopathy
DOG: 100 mg/kg PO BID or 220 mg/kg/day IV
CAT: 50–100 mg/kg/day PO

Carteolol 1% (Ocupress)
Nonselective topical β-blocker for glaucoma
Apply 1 drop to affected eye BID

Cefadroxil (Cefa Tabs, Duricef)
Serious infections
Chapter 85
20 mg/kg PO BID

Cefazolin sodium (Ancef, Kefzol)
Serious infections, endocarditis
Chapters 9, 110
15–30 mg/kg IV/IM TID–QID
Dental surgery
Chapter 27
20–25 mg/kg IV, 1 hr before surgery
Acute abdomen syndrome, osteomyelitis, sepsis
Chapters 35, 37, 79
20 mg/kg IV/IM/SC TID–QID

Cefotaxime (Claforan)
Meningitis
Chapter 24
DOG: 20–40 mg/kg IV/IM/SC TID–QID

Cefoxitin sodium (Mefoxin)
Resistant or serious infections
Chapters 32, 36, 110, 112
DOG: 15–30 mg/kg SC/IM/IV TID–QID
CAT: 22 mg/kg IV TID–QID

Ceftiofur (Naxcel)
Resistant or serious infections
DOG: 2 mg/kg SC SID

Cephalexin (Keflex)
Staphylococcus diskospondylitis, stomatitis
Chapters 24, 27
DOG: 22 mg/kg PO/IM/SC TID

Cephalexin (Keflex) *(continued)*
Borreliosis
    Chapter 78
    DOG: 22 mg/kg PO TID
Serious infections
    Chapters 18, 31, 36, 51, 79, 82, 84, 85, 93, 100, 101
    20–30 mg/kg PO/SC/IM/IV BID–TID

■**Charcoal, activated (Requa, Actidose-Aqua)**
Adsorbent during poisonings
    Chapters 122–128
    Mix 1 g charcoal in 5 ml water, give 10 ml slurry/kg PO

■**Chlorambucil (Leukeran)**
Lymphoplasmacytic stomatitis
    Chapter 27
    DOG: 1–2 mg/m^2 PO QOD
    CAT: 0.25–0.33 mg/kg PO q 3 days
Inflammatory bowel disease
    Chapter 32
    CAT: 1.5 mg/m^2 PO SID–QOD
Chronic lymphocytic leukemia
    Chapter 64
    DOG: a) 0.2 mg/kg PO SID
          b) 15 mg/m^2 PO SID × 5 days, then q 3 wk
    CAT: 2 mg PO QOD
Macroglobulinemia, mast cell tumor
    Chapters 70, 75
    DOG: 0.2 mg/kg PO SID × 10 days, then 0.1 mg/kg
          PO SID, with prednisone
Immune-mediated skin disease
    Chapters 85, 89
    0.1–0.2 mg/kg PO SID–QOD, with prednisone
FIP
    Chapter 110
    CAT: 20 mg/m^2 PO every 2–3 wk

■ Chloramphenicol (Chloromycetin)
Bacterial rickettsial infections
Chapters 17, 52, 84, 100, 111–113
DOG: 25–50 mg/kg IV/PO TID
CAT: 25 mg/kg PO BID

■ Chlorazepate dipotassium (Tranxene-SD)
Anxiolytic drug
Chapter 116
DOG: 0.5–2.0 mg PO q 4–6 h PRN

■ Chlordiazepoxide–clidinium (Librax)
See Clidinium

■ Chlorothiazide (Diuril)
Partial ADH deficiency
Chapter 40
10–40 mg/kg PO BID

■ Chlorpheniramine (Chlor-Trimeton, Novahistine)
Urticaria, antihistamine, allergic skin disease
Chapter 89
DOG: 0.5 mg/kg PO BID–TID
CAT: 2–4 mg PO BID
Excessive grooming, self-trauma, eosinophilic granulomas
Chapters 85, 86
DOG: 4–8 mg PO BID; max = 0.5 mg/kg BID
CAT: 2–4 mg PO SID–BID

■ Chlorpromazine (Thorazine)
Antiemetic
Chapters 30, 32, 35, 37, 110
DOG: a) 0.1–2.2 mg/kg PO SID–QID
b) 0.25–0.5 mg/kg SC/IM SID–QID
c) 0.05–0.1 mg/kg IV TID–QID
CAT: 0.01–0.025 mg/kg IV TID–QID

■ Chlorpropamide (Diabinese)
Partial ADH deficiency
Chapter 40
DOG: 125–250 mg/day PO

■ Cholestyramine (Questran)
Short bowel syndrome, malabsorption
Chapter 32
DOG: 200–300 mg/kg PO BID

■ Chorionic gonadotropin, human (HCG, Follutein, Profasi)
Luteinize a follicular cyst
Chapters 54, 61
DOG: 500–1000 IU IM; repeat in 48 hr
CAT: 250–500 IU IM
Induce ovulation
Chapter 61
DOG: 500–1000 IU SC SID × 2 days, after FSH
CAT: 250 IU IM on days 1 and 2 of estrus

■ Cimetidine (Tagamet)
Esophagitis, gastric ulceration
Chapters 29, 37
DOG: 1–4 mg/kg PO/IV/IM TID–QID
Chronic gastritis, GI tract ulceration, EPI, enteric viruses
Chapters 30–32, 35, 110
DOG: 5–10 mg/kg PO/IV/IM TID–QID
CAT: 5 mg/kg PO/IV TID–QID
Chronic renal failure
Chapter 47
DOG: 4 mg/kg PO/IV/SC BID–TID
Effects of mast cell tumors
Chapters 71, 91
DOG: 4–6 mg/kg PO/IV/SC BID–QID
Protectant, with use of NSAIDs
Chapters 78, 128
DOG: 5–10 mg/kg PO TID

Ciprofloxacin (Cipro)
Osteomyelitis
> Chapter 79
> **DOG:** 11 mg/kg PO BID

Cisapride (not available in USA)
Gastric motility disorders, megacolon
> Chapters 30, 33, 37
> **DOG:** 0.1 mg/kg PO BID–TID or 2.5–5.0 mg PO TID
> **CAT:** 0.3–0.5 mg/kg PO BID–TID or 2.5 mg PO BID–TID

Bladder atony
> Chapter 50
> **DOG:** 0.5 mg/kg PO TID
> **CAT:** 1.25–5.0 mg/cat PO BID–TID

Cisplatin (Platinol)
Chemotherapy, in a protocol
> Chapters 19, 27, 41, 70, 79
> **LARGE DOG:** 60–70 mg/m^2 IV with saline
> **SMALL DOG:** 50–60 mg/m^2 IV with saline

Clarithromycin (Biaxin)
Hepatozoonosis
> **DOG:** 5–10 mg/kg PO BID × 14–21 days

Clemastine (Tavist)
Antihistamine, allergic skin disease
> Chapter 89
> **DOG:** 0.05–0.1 mg/kg PO BID
> **CAT:** 0.67 mg/cat PO BID

Clidinium (Librax)
Irritable colon syndrome
> Chapter 33
> **DOG:** 0.1–0.25 mg/kg PO BID–TID

Clindamycin (Cleocin, Antirobe)
Bronchiectasis
Chapter 17
DOG: 10–12.5 mg/kg PO BID
Protozoal polymyositis/neuritis
Chapters 25, 80
10 mg/kg PO TID–QID
Stomatitis, dental disease
Chapter 27
10 mg/kg PO BID
Toxoplasmosis, prostatitis, hepatozoonosis
Chapters 32, 52, 100, 114
10–20 mg/kg PO/IM BID × 3–6 wk
Babesiosis
Chapter 63
12.5 mg/kg PO BID
Osteomyelitis
Chapter 79
11 mg/kg PO/IM/IV BID–TID
Bacterial folliculitis, cellulitis
Chapter 84
10 mg/kg PO BID

Clofazimine (Lamprene)
Feline leprosy
Chapter 111
CAT: 8 mg/kg PO SID × 6 wk

Clomiphene citrate (Clomid, Serophene)
Antiestrogen agent, male infertility
DOG: 25 mg/kg PO SID

Clomipramine (Anafranil)
Certain behavioral, dermatologic disorders
Chapters 86, 116, 117
DOG: 1–3 mg/kg PO SID–BID, in a protocol
CAT: 0.5 mg/kg PO SID

Clorazepate dipotassium (Tranxene-SD)
Seizures
Chapter 22
DOG: 2 mg/kg PO BID
CAT: 3.75 mg/cat PO BID
Anxiolytic drug
Chapter 116
DOG: 0.5–2 mg/kg PO q 4–6 h

Clotrimazole (Lotrimin, Mycelex)
Candidiasis, fungal rhinitis
Chapters 14, 84
Apply topically as directed

Cloxacillin
Staphylococcus diskospondylitis
Chapter 24
10 mg/kg PO QID

Cobalamin
See Vitamin B$_{12}$

Colchicine (Colchicine, ColBenemid)
Chronic hepatic fibrosis
Chapter 34
DOG: 0.03 mg/kg PO SID

Cortisone acetate (Cortone acetate)
Hypoadrenocorticism
1 mg/kg/day PO/IM

Coumarin (nonanticoagulant form)
Lymphedema
Chapter 67
DOG: 400 mg/kg/day PO

Cyclophosphamide (Cytoxan)

Pulmonary eosinophilic diseases
>Chapter 18
>**DOG:** 50 mg/m^2 PO QOD

Glomerulonephritis, granulomatous urethritis
>Chapters 47, 51
>**DOG:** 2.2 mg/kg or 50 mg/m^2 PO SID × 4 days/wk

Feline mammary cancer
>Chapter 59
>**CAT:** 50–100 mg/m^2 PO, in a protocol with doxorubicin

Immune thrombocytopenia (use with caution)
>Chapter 66
>**DOG:** 2 mg/kg or 50 mg/m^2 PO SID × 4 days/wk × 3–4 wk

Immune hemolytic anemia
>Chapter 63
>50 mg/m^2 or 2 mg/kg PO/IV SID × 4 days/wk

Lymphosarcoma, myeloproliferative disorders, multiple myeloma, as part of a protocol
>Chapters 67, 70, 75
>a) 50 mg/m^2 PO QOD–SID
>b) 250–300 mg/m^2 PO/IV q 3 wk

Autoimmune skin diseases, SLE
>Chapters 74, 89
>**DOG:** 50 mg/m^2 PO SID × 4 days/wk or QOD

Rheumatoid, immune-mediated arthritis
>Chapter 78
>**DOG:** 1.5–2.5 mg/kg PO SID × 4 days/wk

Polymyositis
>Chapter 80
>1–2 mg/kg PO SID × 4 days/wk

FIP
>Chapter 110
>**CAT:** 2 mg/kg PO SID × 4 days/wk, with prednisone

Cyclosporine (Sandimmune, Neoral)

Feline allergic bronchitis
>Chapter 17
>**CAT:** 10 mg/kg PO BID

Perianal fistulas
    Chapter 36
    DOG: 5 mg/kg PO BID
Glomerulonephritis
    Chapter 47
    DOG: 15 mg/kg PO SID
Immune hemolytic anemia
    Chapter 63
    DOG: 10 mg/kg PO SID or dd BID
Sebaceous adenitis, unresponsive atopy
    Chapters 85, 89
    DOG: 5–10 mg/kg PO SID × 5 days, off 2 days, then
        2.5–5 mg/kg PO SID × 5 days, then taper

Cyclosporine (Optimmune)
KCS, pigmentary keratitis, pannus, plasmoma of third eyelid, immune conjunctivitis
    Chapters 94–96
    DOG: Apply ¼ in. to affected eye BID–TID

Cyproheptadine (Periactin)
Allergic bronchitis
    Chapter 17
    CAT: 2 mg PO BID
Appetite stimulant
    Chapters 70, 71, 109
    DOG: 3 mg/kg PO BID–TID
    CAT: 1–2 mg/kg PO SID–BID

Cytosine arabinoside (Cytosar)
Lymphosarcoma, myeloproliferative disorders, as part of a protocol
    Chapter 70
    100 mg/m^2/day IV CRI × 4 days or 300 mg/m^2 SC BID × 2 days

Dacarbazine (DTIC–Dome)
Chemotherapy
    Chapter 70
    DOG: 200 mg/m^2 IV SID × 5 days; repeat cycle q 3 wk

Danazol (Danocrine)
Immune hemolytic anemia, thrombocytopenia
    Chapters 63, 66
    DOG: 2–5 mg/kg PO BID–TID

Dantrolene (Dantrium)
Functional urethral obstruction
    Chapter 50
    DOG: 1–5 mg/kg PO BID–TID
    CAT: 0.5–2 mg/kg PO TID or 1 mg/kg IV
Malignant hyperthermia
    Chapter 80
    DOG: 2–5 mg/kg IV once

Dapsone (Avlosulfon)
Feline mycobacteriosis
    Chapter 111
    CAT: 1 mg/kg PO TID–QID × 4–6 wk
**Familial vasculopathy, cutaneous vasculitis,
subcorneal pustular dermatosis**
    Chapters 82, 85, 89
    DOG: 1 mg/kg PO TID × 14 days, then taper
    CAT: 1 mg/kg PO SID; use with caution

Deferoxamine (Desferal)
Iron toxicity
    Chapter 127
    40 mg/kg IM QID or 15 mg/kg/hr IV (with caution) ×
        1–2 days

Dehydrocholic acid (Decholin)
Cholangitis, cholelithiasis
    DOG: 15 mg/kg PO TID until urine negative for bilirubin

Delmadinone acetate (Tardak) (not available in USA)
Galactorrhea
    Chapter 59
    DOG: 1–1.5 mg/kg SC

Demeclocycline (Declomycin)
Inappropriate ADH secretion
   Chapter 71
   DOG: 3–6 mg/kg PO SID–BID

L-Deprenyl (Anipryl)
Hyperadrenocorticism
   Chapter 44
   DOG: 1 mg/kg PO SID
Cognitive dysfunction
   Chapter 116
   DOG: 1–2 mg/kg PO SID

Desmopressin acetate (DDAVP)
Central diabetes insipidus
   Chapters 40, 46
   DOG: 2–3 drops BID–TID intranasally, conjunctivally
von Willebrand's disease
   Chapter 66
   DOG: 1 µg/kg SC 90 min prior to surgery

Desoxycorticosterone pivalate (DOCP, Percorten pivalate)
Hypoadrenocorticism
   Chapter 44
   DOG: 1–2 mg/kg IM/SC q 25–28 days
   CAT: 12.5 mg IM q 21–28 days

Dexamethasone NaPO$_4$ (Dexate)
Anti-inflammatory
   Chapters 15, 17, 101
   0.2–1.0 mg/kg IV/SC/PO SID–BID
Feline allergic bronchitis
   Chapter 17
   CAT: 0.2–2.2 mg/kg IV/IM
Hydrocephalus
   Chapter 23
   0.05 mg/kg PO BID, taper to QOD

Dexamethasone NaPO$_4$ (Dexate) *(continued)*
Spinal cord trauma
   Chapter 24
   1–2 mg/kg IV
Shock, anaphylaxis, CPR
   Chapters 8, 31, 44, 74
   1–4 mg/kg IV slowly
Hypercalcemia
   Chapters 42, 123
   0.1–0.2 mg/kg IV/SC BID or 0.25 mg/kg SC QID
Juvenile cellulitis
   Chapter 85
   DOG: 0.2 mg/kg PO SID
Immune-mediated skin diseases
   Chapter 89
   CAT: 0.2–0.4 mg/kg PO SID, then taper
Cerebral edema
   Chapters 134, 135
   0.25–2 mg/kg IV, then 0.25–1 mg/kg SC TID–QID in
      tapering doses

Dextran 40 or 70 (Rheomacrodex)
Shock
   Chapters 8, 31, 37, 131
   DOG: 10–20 ml/kg IV or 2 ml/kg/hr IV infusion
   CAT: 5–10 ml/kg IV slowly
Burns, heat prostration
   Chapters 133, 134
   20 ml/kg/day IV in 5% D/W

Dextrose 50%
Hypoglycemia, insulin overdosage
   Chapters 37, 44, 45
   1–2 ml/kg PO or 0.25–1 ml/kg IV

Diazepam (Valium)
Restraint, pain relief
   Chapters 3, 4, 8
   DOG: 0.2–0.6 mg/kg IV
   CAT: 0.1–0.2 mg/kg IV

Seizures
   Chapters 22, 110
   CAT: 2.5 mg PO TID; max = 7.5 mg PO TID
      Rectal administration:
      DOG: 1–3 mg/kg; max = 2 mg/kg/dose if on
            phenobarbital
   CAT: 0.5 mg/kg
Status epilepticus, certain toxicoses
   Chapters 22, 110, 122–130
   a) 0.5–1 mg/kg IV in increments of 5–20 mg, to effect
   b) **DOG:** 0.2–0.5 mg/kg/hr IV in 0.9% NaCl CRI
   c) **CAT:** 0.3 mg/kg/hr IV in 0.9% NaCl CRI
Acquired tremors
   Chapter 23
   0.25 mg/kg PO TID–QID
Scotty cramps
   Chapter 23
   0.5 mg/kg PO TID
Preanesthetic
   Chapter 31
   DOG: 0.25–0.50 mg/kg IV slowly, with ketamine,
         oxymorphone, hydromorphone
Sedation
   Chapters 37, 80, 134
   DOG: a) 0.5–2.2 mg/kg PO PRN
         b) 0.5 mg/kg IV to effect
   CAT: 0.2–0.6 mg/kg IV
Functional urethral obstruction, FUS
   Chapters 49, 50
   DOG: 2–10 mg PO SID–QID
   CAT: 1–2.5 mg PO SID–QID or 0.5 mg/kg IV
Appetite stimulant
   Chapter 71
   CAT: 0.05–0.15 mg/kg IV SID–QOD or 1 mg PO SID
Urine marking, anxiety, psychogenic alopecia
   Chapter 86
   DOG: 0.25–1.1 mg/kg PO BID
   CAT: 0.2 mg/kg PO BID
Vertigo
   Chapter 106
   DOG: 0.1–0.2 mg/kg PO SID–BID

Diazepam (Valium) *(continued)*
Certain behavioral disorders
    Chapters 116, 117
    DOG: 0.5–2.0 mg/kg PO q 4–6 h PRN
    CAT: 1–2 mg/cat PO SID–BID

Diazoxide (Proglycem)
Hypoglycemia
    Chapters 45, 71
    DOG: 5–13 mg/kg PO BID–TID; max = 40 mg/kg/day

Dichlorphenamide (Daranide)
Glaucoma
    DOG: 2–4 mg/kg PO BID–TID
    CAT: 1 mg/kg PO BID–TID

Diclofenac 0.1% (Voltaren)
Anterior uveitis
    Chapter 97
    Apply 1 drop to affected eye BID–QID

Dicyclomine (Bentyl)
Decrease bladder contractility
    Chapter 50
    DOG: 10 mg PO TID

Diethylcarbamazine (Filaribits)
Heartworm prophylaxis
    Chapter 12
    DOG: 6.6 mg/kg PO SID

Diethylstilbestrol (DES, Stilphostrol)
Hormone-responsive incontinence
    Chapter 50
    DOG: 0.1–1 mg PO SID × 5 days, then q 5–14 days
Induce estrus
    Chapter 60
    DOG: 5 mg PO SID × 6–9 days

Digoxin (Lanoxin)
Congestive heart failure, supraventricular tachyarrhythmias
> Chapters 7, 9, 10
> **DOG:** 0.005–0.01 mg/kg PO BID or 0.22 mg/m² PO BID
> **CAT:** 0.005–0.008 mg/kg PO QOD–SID or 0.031 mg PO QOD–SID

Digoxin immune Fab (Digibind)
Digoxin toxicity
> Chapter 7
> **DOG:** 40 mg IV (over 30 min) per mg digoxin ingested

Dihydrotachysterol (DHT Tablets)
Hypocalcemia
> Chapter 42
> 0.02 mg/kg/day PO × 3 days, then 0.01–0.02 mg/kg PO SID–QOD

1,25-Dihydroxyvitamin D₃
> *See* Calcitriol

Diltiazem (Cardizem)
Hypertrophic cardiomyopathy, supraventricular tachyarrhythmias
> Chapters 7, 9, 10
> **DOG:** 0.5–1.5 mg/kg PO TID
> **CAT:** 1.5–2.4 mg/kg PO BID–TID

Dimenhydrinate (Dramamine)
Motion sickness
> **DOG:** 25–50 mg PO SID–TID
> **CAT:** 12.5 mg PO SID–TID

Dimercaprol (BAL)
Arsenic toxicosis
> Chapters 122, 127
> 3–5 mg/kg IM QID × 5 days

Dimethyl sulfoxide 40% (DMSO)
Spinal cord trauma
Chapter 24
DOG: 1 g/kg IV in 5% D/W SID × 3–4 days

Diminazene aceturate (Berenil) (not available in USA)
Babesiosis, trypanosomiasis
Chapter 63
DOG: 3.5 mg/kg IM once

Dioctyl sulfosuccinate (Colace, Surfak, Docusate)
Stool softener
Chapter 33
SMALL DOG, CAT: 25 mg PO SID–BID
MEDIUM/LARGE DOG: 50–100 mg PO SID–BID

Diosmin
Lymphedema
DOG: 3 g/day PO

Diphenhydramine HCl (Benadryl)
Rhinitis
Chapter 14
DOG: 2–4 mg/kg PO TID
Counteract effects of mast cell tumors
Chapters 71, 91
1 mg/kg IM BID–TID or 2–4 mg/kg PO TID
Anaphylaxis, urticaria, angioneurotic edema
Chapter 74
1–2 mg/kg IM/IV slowly
Antipruritic, allergic skin disease
Chapter 89
DOG: 2 mg/kg PO/IM BID–TID
Nicotinic receptor overload
Chapters 122, 124
DOG: 1–4 mg/kg PO TID

Diphenoxylate HCl (Lomotil)
Acute colitis, irritable colon syndrome
Chapter 33
DOG: 0.05–0.1 mg/kg PO TID–QID
CAT: 0.063 mg/kg PO TID
Antidiarrheal
DOG: 2.5 mg PO BID–QID
CAT: 0.6–1.2 mg PO BID–TID

Diphenylthiocarbazone (Dithizone)
Thallium toxicosis
Chapter 122
50–70 mg/kg PO TID

Disodium EDTA
See EDTA

Dobutamine HCl (Dobutrex)
Inotropic agent
Chapters 8, 74, 131, 134
DOG: 2–25 µg/kg/min IV infusion
CAT: 1–2 µg/kg/min IV infusion
Pulmonary hypertension
Chapter 18
DOG: 5–7 µg/kg/min IV

Dopamine HCl (Inotropin)
Inotropic agent
Chapters 8, 31, 131, 134
2–25 µg/kg/min IV infusion
Pulmonary hypertension
Chapter 18
DOG: 5–7 µg/kg/min IV
Renal vasodilator: acute renal failure
Chapters 47, 134
1–10 µg/kg/min IV infusion in 5% D/W

Dorzolamide 2% (Trusopt)
Glaucoma
> Chapter 98
> 1 drop to affected eye BID–TID

Doxapram (Dopram)
Respiratory stimulant
> 5–10 mg/kg IV

Doxepin (Sinequan)
Acral lick dermatitis
> Chapter 86
> **DOG:** 3–5 mg/kg PO BID; max = 150 mg BID
> **CAT:** 0.5–1.0 mg/cat PO SID–BID

Doxorubicin (Adriamycin)
Chemotherapy
> Chapters 41, 59, 67, 70, 79
> **DOG:** a) 25–30 mg/m² IV in 150 ml 5% D/W q 2–9 wk;
>   max cumulative dose = 180 mg/m²
>   b) **SMALL DOG:** 1 mg/kg IV slowly
> **CAT:** a) 20–30 mg/m² IV q 3 wk; max cumulative dose =
>   50 mg/m²
>   b) 1 mg/kg IV slowly

Doxycycline (Vibramycin, Doryx)
Rickettsial infections, leptospirosis, tuberculosis, borreliosis, hepatozoonosis
> Chapters 16, 17, 27, 47, 63, 66, 78, 100, 111–114
> **DOG:** Acute disease: 5–10 mg/kg PO/IV BID × 10–14 days
>   Chronic disease: 10 mg/kg PO SID × 7–21 days
> **CAT:** 2.5–5 mg/kg PO BID
Erosive polyarthritis
> Chapter 78
> **DOG:** 10 mg/kg PO BID

■ Edrophonium Cl (Tensilon, Enlon)
Tensilon test
Chapter 25
DOG: 0.2–5 mg IV; max = 5 mg
PUPPIES: 0.1–0.5 mg IV

■ EDTA, disodium 1%
Calcium keratopathy
Chapters 95, 96
1 drop topically BID–TID

■ Eicosapentanoic acid
See Essential fatty acids

■ Enalapril (Enacard, Vasotec)
Hypertension, heart failure, valvular insufficiency
Chapters 9, 10, 47
DOG: 0.25–0.5 mg/kg PO SID–BID
CAT: 0.25–0.5 mg/kg PO SID–QOD

■ Enilconazole (not available in USA)
Nasal aspergillosis
Chapter 14
Administer 5% solution topically × 2–3 Rx

■ Enrofloxacin (Baytril)
Intracranial infections
Chapter 23
CAT: 5 mg/kg PO BID × 14 days
Diskospondylitis, prostatitis, osteomyelitis
Chapters 24, 52, 79
DOG: 5–15 mg/kg PO BID
Sepsis
Chapter 31
DOG: 10–20 mg/kg IV SID

Enrofloxacin (Baytril) *(continued)*
Resistant infections, mycoplasmal or leptospiral infections
    Chapters 16, 24, 32, 47, 84, 100, 110–112
    DOG: 2.5–5 mg/kg PO/SC/IV BID
    CAT: 1–2.5 mg/kg PO BID
Rickettsial infections
    Chapter 113
    DOG: 3–5 mg/kg PO/IM BID × 7–14 days

Ephedrine (Mudrane GG, Quadrinal)
Bronchodilator
    DOG: 5–15 mg PO BID–TID
    CAT: 2–5 mg PO BID–TID
Urethral sphincter incompetence
    Chapter 50
    DOG: 1.2 mg/kg PO TID
    CAT: 2–4 mg PO TID

Epinephrine (Adrenalin)
Cardiac arrest
    Chapter 8
    1:10,000 soln: 0.1 ml/kg IV/IO or 0.2–0.4 ml/kg IT
Anaphylaxis
    Chapter 74
    1:10,000 soln:
        At site: 0.2–0.5 ml SC/IM
        IV: 0.5–1 ml; repeat in 30 min
        Maximum: 2 ml/dose

Epsiprantel (Cestex)
Dipylidium, Taenia
    Chapters 32, 33
    DOG: 5 mg/kg PO
    CAT: 2.5 mg/kg PO

Ergocalciferol
    See Vitamin D$_2$

Erythromycin (E-Mycin, Ilotycin)
Campylobacter, salmonellosis, mastitis, prostatitis
Chapters 32, 52, 111, 112
DOG: 8–40 mg/kg PO BID–TID
CAT: 10–15 mg/kg PO TID
Gastric motility disorders, megacolon
Chapters 30, 33
DOG: 0.5–1.0 mg/kg PO TID
Bacterial folliculitis
Chapter 84
10–15 mg/kg PO TID

Erythropoietin (Epogen)
Anemia from renal failure
Chapters 47, 63
50–150 U/kg SC 2–3 times/wk PRN
Myelodysplastic disorders
Chapter 65
DOG: 100 U/kg SC QOD × 10 days

Esmolol (Brevibloc)
Supraventricular tachycardia
Chapter 7
250–500 µg/kg slowly IV or CRI of 50–200 µg/kg/min IV

Essential fatty acids
Atopy, fatty acid deficiency
Chapters 89, 90, 120
DOG: Dermcaps: 1 cap/10–20 kg or 1 ml/10 kg PO SID
EFA-2 plus: 2.5 ml/5 kg PO SID
Pet-Tabs/FA granules: 1 tsp/5 kg PO SID

Ethacrynate sodium (Edecrin)
Diuretic: pulmonary edema
0.2–0.4 mg/kg IV/IM q 4–12 h

Ethambutol (Myambutol)
Tuberculosis
DOG: 15 mg/kg PO SID

Ethanol 20%
Ethylene glycol toxicosis
Chapters 122, 127
DOG: 5.5 ml/kg IV q 4 h × 5 Rx, then q 6 h × 4 Rx
CAT: 5 ml/kg IV q 6 h × 5 Rx, then q 8 h × 4 Rx

Etidronate disodium (Didronel)
Hypercalcemia
Chapters 42, 71
DOG: 10–30 mg/kg/day PO/IV × 1–2 Rx

Etodolac (Etogesic)
Musculoskeletal pain or inflammation
Chapters 78, 79
DOG: 10–15 mg/kg PO SID

Famotidine (Pepcid)
Gastric irritation or ulcers, esophagitis, enteric viruses
Chapters 15, 17, 29–34, 37, 47, 91, 110
DOG: 0.5–1 mg/kg PO/SC SID–BID

Felbamate (Felbatol)
Seizures
Chapter 22
DOG: 20 mg/kg PO TID; max = 3000 mg/day

Fenbendazole (Panacur)
Oslerus, Capillaria, Aelurostrongylus
Chapters 14, 16, 18, 47
DOG: 50 mg/kg PO SID × 3–30 days
CAT: 25 mg/kg PO BID × 3–10 days
Hookworms, whipworms, roundworms, *Taenia*
Chapters 32, 33
DOG: 50 mg/kg (1 ml/2 kg) PO SID × 3 days; repeat in
3 wk

Paragonimus, **pancreatic flukes**
> Chapters 18, 35
> **DOG:** 50 mg/kg PO SID × 3–6 days
> **CAT:** 30 mg/kg PO SID × 3–6 days

Crenosoma vulpis, *Giardia canis*, **trichomoniasis**
> Chapter 114
> **DOG:** 50 mg/kg PO SID × 3–7 days

▪ Fentanyl transdermal patch (Duragesic)
Analgesia
> Chapters 70, 79
> **DOG:** 3–5 µg/kg q 3 days

▪ Fentanyl
Pain control
> Chapter 37
> **DOG:** 3 µg/kg IV, then CRI of 3–6 µg/kg/hr IV
> **CAT:** 3 µg/kg IV, then CRI of 1–5 µg/kg/hr IV

▪ Ferric cyanoferrate (Prussian blue)
Thallium toxicosis
> Chapter 122
> 100 mg/kg PO TID

▪ Ferrous sulfate (Feosol, Iberet)
Dietary iron supplement, iron deficiency anemia
> Chapter 63
> **DOG:** 100–300 mg PO SID
> **CAT:** 50–100 mg PO SID

▪ Finasteride (Propecia)
Benign prostatic hyperplasia
> Chapter 52
> **DOG:** 5 mg PO SID

▪ Fipronil (Frontline, Topspot)
Ear mites
> Chapter 87
> Apply 2 drops in each ear; repeat in 2 wk

Fipronil (Frontline, Topspot) *(continued)*
Sarcoptic mange, cheyletiellosis, trombiculiasis
   Chapter 87
   Apply topically 1–2 Rx, 2–4 wk apart
Flea adulticide
   Chapter 87
   Apply topically once monthly as directed

Fluconazole (Diflucan)
Fungal rhinitis, cystitis and stomatitis, systemic mycoses
   Chapters 14, 27, 32, 49, 100, 109
   DOG: 1.25–2.5 mg/kg PO/IV BID or 2.5–5.0 mg/kg PO SID
   CAT: 50 mg PO BID or 2.5–5 mg/kg PO/IV SID

Flucytosine (Ancobon)
Cryptococcus
   Chapters 14, 49, 109
   DOG: 25–50 mg/kg PO QID
   CAT: 100 mg PO QID

Fludrocortisone (Florinef)
Hypoadrenocorticism
   Chapter 44
   0.02 mg/kg/day PO

Flunixin meglumine (Banamine)
Acral lick dermatitis
   Chapter 86
   DOG: mix 3 ml in one bottle Synotic, apply topically
          BID–TID
Antiprostaglandin effects for ocular disease
   DOG: 0.5 mg/kg IV SID–BID × 1–2 Rx
Shock
   Chapter 131
   DOG: 1 mg/kg IV once
   CAT: 0.5 mg/kg IV once

5-Fluorouracil (Efudex)
Colonic adenocarcinoma, in a protocol
> DOG: 150 mg/m^2 IV once weekly

Fluoxetine (Prozac)
Certain behavioral, dermatologic disorders
> Chapters 86, 116, 117
> DOG: 1 mg/kg PO SID
> CAT: 0.5 mg/kg PO SID

Fluoxymesterone (Android F, Halotestin)
Testosterone responsive dermatosis
> DOG: 0.5 mg/kg PO QOD × 12 wk; max = 30 mg/day

Flurbiprofen 0.03% (Ocufen)
Anterior uveitis
> Chapter 97
> Apply topically BID–QID to affected eye

Folic acid (Feosol Plus)
Dietary supplement, folate deficiency
> Chapters 32, 63
> DOG: 1–5 mg/day PO/SC or 4–10 μg/kg/day PO, then
> weekly
> CAT: 2.5 mg/day PO
Supplement to pyrimethamine
> 1 mg/day PO

Follicle-stimulating hormone (FSH-p; pregnant mare serum, PMS)
Male hypogonadism
> DOG: 25 mg SC once weekly or 1 mg/kg IM QOD
Induction of estrus
> DOG: 20 IU/kg SC SID × 10 days, then 500 IU HCG SID ×
> 2 days
> CAT: FSH-p = 2 mg IM SID × 5 days

Furazolidone (Furoxone)
Giardia, coccidia
> Chapters 32, 114
> > 4–10 mg/kg PO SID–BID × 5–7 days

Furosemide (Lasix, Salix)
Diuresis: heart failure
> Chapters 8–10
> > **DOG:** 2–4 mg/kg IV/IM/SC BID–QID, then taper to 1–2 mg/kg PO SID–BID
> > **CAT:** 1–3 mg/kg IV/IM/SC BID–TID, then taper

Diuresis: pulmonary edema
> Chapters 18, 132
> > **DOG:** 2–4 mg/kg IV/IM/PO q 4–12 h
> > **CAT:** 0.5–2 mg/kg IV TID

Hydrocephalus, brain edema
> Chapter 23
> > **DOG:** 1–2 mg/kg PO BID

Diuresis: ascites from hepatic failure
> Chapter 34
> > 0.25–0.5 mg/kg PO/SC SID–BID

Diuresis: hypercalcemia
> Chapters 42, 71, 123
> > 1–2 mg/kg IV/IM/SC/PO BID–TID

Hypertension
> Chapter 47
> > 1 mg/kg PO SID–BID

Institute diuresis in acute renal failure, certain toxicoses
> Chapters 47, 122, 134
> > 2–6 mg/kg IV TID PRN or 0.1–1.0 mg/kg/hr IV

Gabapentin (Neurontin)
Seizures
> Chapter 22
> > **DOG:** 10–20 mg/kg PO TID

Gallium nitrate
Hypercalcemia
> Chapter 71
> **DOG:** 2.5 µg/kg IV SID × 5 days

Gamma globulin, human (Iveegam)
Immune hemolytic anemia
> Chapter 63
> **DOG:** 0.5–1.5 g/kg IV over 12 hr

Gentamicin (Gentocin)
Serious bacterial infections, osteomyelitis
> Chapters 9, 24, 31, 79, 110, 111
> 5–6 mg/kg IV/SC/IM SID

Glipizide (Glucotrol)
Feline diabetes mellitus
> Chapter 43
> **CAT:** 2.5–5 mg PO BID

Glucagon (Glucagon)
Induce gastric hypomotility
> Chapter 4
> **DOG:** 0.1–0.35 mg IV
> **CAT:** 0.1 mg IV

Transient improvement in hypoglycemia
> Chapters 45, 71
> **DOG: a)** 0.03 mg/kg IV/IM/SC
>   **b)** 50 ng/kg IV once, then CRI of 10–40 ng/kg/min IV

Glucose 40% ophthalmic ointment
Corneal edema, nonhealing erosions
> Chapter 96
> Apply ⅛ in. topically 2–6 times daily

Glycerin
Acute glaucoma
> Chapter 98
> **DOG:** 1–2 g/kg PO × 1–2 Rx

Glyceryl guaiacolate (Geocolate)
Muscle relaxation during certain toxicoses
    Chapters 122–129
    110 mg/kg IV PRN

Glyceryl monoacetate
Sodium fluoroacetate toxicosis
    Chapter 122
    0.55 mg/kg IM hourly to 2–4 mg/kg

Glycopyrrolate (Robinul)
Sinus bradycardia, heart block
    Chapter 7
    0.005–0.01 mg/kg IV/IM or 0.01–0.02 mg/kg SC PRN
Hypersialism
    Chapter 28
    0.01 mg/kg SC PRN
Preanesthetic
    0.01–0.02 mg/kg SC/IM

Gonadotropin-releasing hormone (Cystorelin)
Luteinize an ovarian follicular cyst
    Chapters 54, 61
    DOG: 50–100 µg IM SID × 1–3 Rx
    CAT: 25 µg IM
Stimulate descent of inguinal testis
    DOG: 50–100 µg IV/SC weekly for 2 Rx
Poor libido in male dogs
    Chapter 60
    DOG: 1–2 µg/kg IM 1 hour before breeding
Induce ovulation
    Chapters 57, 61
    DOG: 50 µg IV or 2.2 µg/kg IM
    CAT: 25 µg IM after mating or before artificial
        insemination

Granulocyte colony-stimulating factor (Neupogen)
Neutropenia
Chapters 64, 73
2.5–10.0 µg/kg/day SC × 3–5 days

Griseofulvin (Fulvicin, Grisactin)
Dermatomycoses
Chapter 84
Microsized: 10–30 mg/kg PO BID × 12 wk
Ultramicrosized: 2.5–5.0 mg/kg PO SID–BID × 12 wk

Growth hormone (Protropin, Bovine GH)
Pituitary dwarfism
Chapter 40
DOG: 0.1 IU/kg SC SID 3 days/wk × 4–6 wk
Adult hyposomatotropism
Chapter 88
DOG: 0.15 IU/kg SC twice weekly for 6 wk

Halothane (Fluothane)
Anesthesia
Induction: 3%
Maintenance: 0.5–1.5%

Heparin
Arterial thromboembolism, thrombophlebitis
Chapters 10, 18
DOG: 200 U/kg IV, then 75–200 U/kg SC TID–QID
CAT: 100 U/kg SC TID
DIC
Chapters 37, 63, 133, 134
75–100 U/kg SC/IV TID–QID or 150–200 U/kg SC QID

Hetastarch (Hespan)
Shock, hypoproteinemia, CPR
Chapters 8, 32, 37, 110, 131, 133, 134, 136
DOG: 10–20 ml/kg/day IV
CAT: 10–15 ml/kg IV

▪ Human gamma globulin
See Gamma globulin, human

▪ Hydralazine (Apresoline)
Vasodilator: heart failure
Chapter 9
DOG: 0.5–2 mg/kg PO BID
CAT: 2–5 mg PO BID
Hypertension
Chapter 47
DOG: 0.5 mg/kg PO BID
CAT: 2.5 mg PO BID
Acute arterial thromboembolism
DOG: 0.5–2 mg/kg PO/IM BID
CAT: 2.5 mg PO BID

▪ Hydrochlorothiazide (HydroDiuril)
Diuretic: pulmonary edema
Chapter 9
2–4 mg/kg PO SID–BID
Nephrogenic diabetes insipidus
Chapter 40
0.5–1.0 mg/kg PO BID
Hypoglycemia
Chapter 71
DOG: 2–4 mg/kg PO BID, with diazoxide
Hypertension
Chapter 47
DOG: 0.5–5 mg/kg PO BID
CAT: 1–2 mg/kg PO BID

▪ Hydrocodone bitartrate (Hycodan)
Cough suppressant, acral lick dermatitis
Chapters 15–17, 86, 112
DOG: 0.22 mg/kg PO BID–QID
Feline compulsive disorders
Chapter 117
CAT: 1.25–2.5 mg PO SID–BID

Hydrocortisone sodium succinate (Solu-Cortef)
Shock
  10 mg/kg IV
Feline asthma
  CAT: 1–3 mg/kg IV

Hydrogen peroxide 3%
Emetic
  Chapter 122
  1.5 ml/kg PO × 1–2 Rx

Hydromorphone (Dilaudid, Hydromorphone)
Preanesthetic, sedation
  Chapters 15, 17, 31
  DOG: 0.05–0.2 mg/kg IV
Analgesic
  Chapters 31, 37, 79
  DOG: 0.1–0.2 mg/kg IV
  CAT: 0.02–0.1 mg/kg IV

Hydroxyethyl starch
  See Hetastarch

Hydroxyurea (Hydrea)
Primary polycythemia, thrombocytosis
  Chapters 63, 70
  DOG: a) 15 mg/kg PO SID until PCV normalizes
      b) 80 mg/kg PO q 3 days
  CAT: 25 mg/kg PO 3 times weekly
Eosinophilic leukemia
  Chapter 65
  CAT: 40 mg/kg/day PO × 7 days, then QOD, then q 3 days
Chronic granulocytic leukemia, basophilic leukemia
  Chapter 65
  DOG: a) 20–25 mg/kg or 0.5 g/m^2 PO BID × 4–6 wk, then
      50 mg/kg PO twice weekly
      b) 50 mg/kg PO SID × 14 days, then QOD, then
      q 3 days

Hydroxyzine (Atarax)
Antihistamine, allergic skin disease, urticaria
Chapters 86, 89, 93
DOG: 2.2 mg/kg PO BID–TID
CAT: 2.2 mg/kg PO BID

Hyoscyamine (Levsin)
Irritable bowel syndrome
Chapter 33
DOG: 0.003–0.006 mg/kg PO BID–TID

Hypertonic saline (7.5%)
Shock, CPR
Chapters 8, 31
4–5 ml/kg IV slowly; max = 10 ml/kg
Hyponatremia, severe
Chapter 71
5–20 ml/kg IV

Idoxuridine 0.1% (Herplex)
Ocular herpesvirus infection
Chapters 94, 96, 112
Apply topically 4–8 times daily

Ifosfamide (Ifex)
Lymphosarcoma
Chapter 70
DOG: 350–375 mg/m^2 IV, with mesna, q 2–3 wk

Imidacloprid (Advantage)
Flea adulticide
Chapter 87
Apply topically once monthly, as directed

Imidocarb dipropionate (Imizol) (not available in USA)

Babesiosis, ehrlichiosis, cytanzoonosis, hepatozoonosis

Chapters 63, 113, 114

DOG: 5–7.5 mg/kg IM/SC; repeat in 14 days

CAT: 2–5 mg/kg IM once; repeat in 14 days

Imipenem (Primaxin)

Septicemia

Chapter 32

DOG: 2–7 mg/kg IV/IM TID

Imipramine (Tofranil)

Urethral sphincter incompetence

Chapter 50

DOG: 5–15 mg PO BID or 0.5–1 mg/kg PO TID

CAT: 2.5–5 mg PO BID–TID

Acral lick dermatitis

Chapter 86

DOG: 2–4 mg/kg PO SID

Insulin, NPH

Diabetes mellitus

Chapter 43

0.5 U/kg SC BID

Insulin, PZI

Diabetes mellitus

Chapter 43

CAT: 0.5 U/kg SC BID

Insulin, regular

Diabetic ketoacidosis

Chapter 43

DOG: a) 0.2 U/kg IM then 0.1 U/kg IM hourly until glucose > 250 mg/dl

b) 2.2 U/kg in 250 ml 0.9% NaCl IV as CRI

Insulin, regular *(continued)*
Hyperkalemia with cardiotoxicity
Chapters 44, 47
DOG: 0.05–0.25 U/kg IV with 1–2 g of glucose per unit

Insulin, Ultralente
Diabetes mellitus
Chapter 43
CAT: 0.5 U/kg SC SID

Interferon, human recombinant (Alferon, Intron, Roferon-A)
FeLV, FIP
Chapters 110, 112
CAT: 30 U PO SID on alternating weeks
Mycosis fungoides
Chapter 91
$1.0–1.5 \times 10^6$ U/m^2 SC 3 times weekly

Iohexol (Omnipaque)
Myelography
Chapter 4
0.3–0.45 ml/kg

Iopamidol (Isovue-200)
Myelography
Chapter 4
0.3–0.45 ml/kg

Ipecac syrup
Induce vomiting
Chapter 122
1–2 ml/kg PO

Ipronidazole
Giardiasis
DOG: 126 mg/L water PO ad libitum × 7 days

Iron dextran (INFeD injection)
Iron deficiency anemia
  Chapter 63
  DOG: 10–20 mg/kg SC

Isoflurane (Forane, AErrane)
Anesthesia
  Induction: 4–5%
  Maintenance: 1.5–2.5%

Isoniazid (Rifamate, Rifater)
Tuberculosis
  10–20 mg/kg PO SID

Isoproterenol (Isuprel)
Bradycardia, heart block
  Chapter 7
  0.01–0.02 µg/kg/min IV as CRI of 0.2–0.5 mg in 250 ml
    5% D/W
Feline asthma
  CAT: 0.2 mg in 100 ml 5% D/W IV TID to effect or
      0.004–0.006 mg IM q 30 min PRN

Isosorbide dinitrate (Isordil)
Vasodilator
  Chapter 9
  DOG: 0.2–1.0 mg/kg PO BID

Isotretinoin (Accutane)
**Sebaceous adenitis or hyperplasia, schnauzer
comedo syndrome, spiculosis**
  Chapters 82, 85, 88, 91
  DOG: 1–3 mg/kg PO SID–BID
  CAT: 5–10 mg/day PO
Mycosis fungoides
  Chapter 91
  DOG: 3–4 mg/kg/day PO
  CAT: 10 mg/day PO

■ Itraconazole (Sporanox)

Systemic mycoses, dermatophytosis, protothecosis, fungal stomatitis or otitis

Chapters 14, 27, 32, 84, 88, 100, 105, 106, 109

DOG: 5 mg/kg PO SID–BID × 2–12 mo

CAT: 5–10 mg/kg PO SID–BID

■ Ivermectin (Heartgard)

Heartworm prophylaxis

Chapter 12

DOG: 6–12 µg/kg PO once monthly

CAT: 24 µg/kg PO once monthly

Microfilaricide

Chapter 12

DOG: 50 µg/kg PO, repeat in 10 days

CAT: 24 µg/kg PO

Pneumonyssus, Capillaria, Oslerus, Strongyloides, Aelurostrongylus

Chapters 14, 16, 18, 32, 47

DOG: 0.2–0.3 mg/kg PO/SC; repeat in 3 wk (Do not use this dosage in collies or shelties.)

CAT: 0.2 mg/kg PO once

Intracranial *Cuterebra* infection

Chapter 23

0.4 mg/kg SC SID × 3 days (Not to be used in collies or shelties.)

Spirocercosis

DOG: 0.2 mg/kg PO once (Not to be used in collies or shelties.)

Cheyletiellosis; notoedric, otodectic, and sarcoptic mange; pediculosis

Chapters 87, 93

DOG: 0.2–0.3 mg/kg PO/SC; repeat in 2 wk (Not to be used in collies or shelties.)

CAT: 0.2–0.4 mg/kg SC; repeat in 2 wk (Not approved for use in cats.)

Demodicosis
Chapters 87, 93
DOG: 0.05 mg/kg PO on day 1, then increase by 0.05 mg/kg daily until reaching 0.4–0.6 mg/kg PO SID × 30 days (Do not use in collie-type, English, or Australian sheepdogs.)

Ivermectin 0.01% otic solution (Acarexx)
Ear mites
Chapter 87
Apply 0.5 ml twice, 2 wk apart

Kaolin/pectin (Kaopectate)
GI tract protectant
Chapters 122, 126
1–2 ml/kg PO BID–QID

Ketamine HCl (Ketaject, Ketamine)
Restraint
Chapters 3, 4
CAT: a) 0.2–0.6 mg/kg IV, with diazepam or acetylpromazine
b) 2–4 mg/kg IV
Anesthesia, sedation
DOG: 6–10 mg/kg IV
CAT: 22–33 mg/kg IM or 2.2–4.4 mg/kg IV
Preanesthetic
Chapter 31
DOG: 2.5–5.5 mg/kg IV, with diazepam

Ketoconazole (Nizoral)
Systemic, oral, and cutaneous mycoses;
prototheocosis; fungal otitis
Chapters 14, 27, 32, 84, 88, 100, 109
DOG: 5–15 mg/kg PO BID
CAT: 10–15 mg/kg PO SID–BID
Hyperadrenocorticism
Chapter 44
DOG: 7.5–15 mg/kg PO BID

Ketoconazole (Nizoral) *(continued)*
Malassezia **otitis**
    Chapters 105, 106
    DOG: 5–10 mg/kg PO SID
Leishmaniasis
    10 mg/kg PO TID × 3 wk

Lactulose (Enulose, Cholac)
Hepatic encephalopathy, stool softener
    Chapters 23, 33, 34
    0.25–0.5 ml/kg (2–10 ml) PO TID–QID until feces are soft

Latanoprost 0.005% (Xalatan)
Glaucoma
    Chapter 98
    1 drop to affected eye SID–BID

Levamisole (Ripercol, Tramisol)
Oslerus, Capillaria
    Chapters 14, 18
    DOG: 8–10 mg/kg PO SID × 5–30 days
Recurrent bacterial folliculitis
    Chapter 84
    DOG: 2.2 mg/kg PO QOD

Levobunolol 0.25%, 0.5% (Betagen)
Nonselective β-blocker for glaucoma
    Apply 1 drop to affected eye SID–BID

Lidocaine
Ventricular arrhythmias
    Chapters 7, 8, 10, 31, 122
    DOG: a) 1–4 mg/kg IV bolus up to a total dose of 8 mg/kg
            in 10 min
        b) 25–80 µg/kg/min IV as CRI
    CAT: a) 0.25–0.75 mg/kg IV slow bolus
        b) 10–40 µg/kg/min IV as CRI

Lime sulfur suspension (Lym Dip)
Sarcoptic and notoedric mange, dermatophytosis, feline demodicosis
Chapters 84, 87
DOG: 1:20 dilution
CAT: 1:40 dilution (4 oz/gal water)
Dip, air-dry; repeat weekly × 6 wk

Lime water
Alkaline gastric lavage
Chapter 122
5 ml/kg PO

Lincomycin (Lincocin)
Mastitis
15 mg/kg PO TID × 21 days
Bacterial folliculitis, blepharitis
Chapters 84, 93
20 mg/kg PO BID

Liothyronine, T$_3$
See Triiodothyronine

Lisinopril (Prinivil)
Heart failure
Chapter 9
DOG: 0.5 mg/kg PO SID

Lithium carbonate (Eskalith, Lithobid)
Cyclic neutropenia, pancytopenia
Chapters 64, 73
DOG: 11 mg/kg PO SID–BID
Drug-induced thrombocytopenia
Chapter 66
DOG: 11 mg/kg PO BID
Refractory, inappropriate ADH secretion
Chapter 71
DOG: 25 mg/kg PO SID

Lomotil (diphenoxylate HCl with atropine)
Antidiarrheal
> **DOG:** 2.5 mg PO BID–TID

Lomustine (CeeNu)
Brain tumors, mast cell tumor, lymphoma rescue
> Chapter 70
> **DOG:** 50–90 mg/m^2 PO q 4–6 wk
> **CAT:** 50–60 mg/m^2 PO q 6 wk

Loperamide (Imodium)
Antidiarrheal, acute colitis
> Chapters 32, 33
> **DOG:** 0.08–0.2 mg/kg PO BID–QID
> **CAT:** 0.04 mg/kg PO SID–BID; use with caution

Lufenuron (Program)
Dermatophytosis
> Chapter 84
> 50–100 mg/kg PO q 14 days × 2 Rx, then once monthly

Flea growth inhibitor
> Chapter 87
> **DOG:** 10 mg/kg PO once monthly
> **CAT:** 30 mg/kg PO once monthly

L-Lysine
Ocular herpesvirus
> Chapters 94, 96, 112
> **CAT:** 250–500 mg PO SID–BID

Lysine-8 vasopressin (Diapid)
Central diabetes insipidus
> Chapter 40
> 1–2 sprays in each nostril SID–TID

Magnesium hydroxide (Milk of Magnesia)
Antacid for certain toxicoses
> Chapter 127
> 1–15 ml PO SID–BID

Magnesium sulfate
Serum magnesium deficit
    Chapter 43
    1 mEq/kg/day IV

Mannitol 20%
Cerebral edema, acute renal failure, diuresis
    Chapters 8, 23, 24, 47, 122, 134
    0.5–1 g/kg IV slowly
Acute glaucoma
    Chapter 98
    0.5–2 g/kg IV slowly

Meclizine (Bonine)
Motion sickness, urticaria
    Chapters 23, 106
    DOG: 1–4 mg/kg PO SID or 0.5 mg/kg PO BID
    CAT: 1–2 mg/kg PO SID

Meclofenamic acid (Arquel)
Degenerative joint disease
    Chapter 78
    DOG: 1.1 mg/kg PO SID × 4–7 days, then 0.5 mg/kg

Medium-chain triglycerides (MCT Oil, Portagen)
Chylothorax
    1–2 ml/kg/day PO
Primary lymphangiectasis, EPI
    Chapter 35
    0.5–1 oz/10 kg PO dd TID–QID; max = 1 tbsp per meal
    or 1–2.2 ml/kg/day PO with food

Medroxyprogesterone acetate (Depo-Provera, Provera)
Aggressive masculine behavior
    DOG: 10 mg/kg IM/SC PRN

Medroxyprogesterone acetate (Depo-Provera, Provera) *(continued)*
Urine marking, anxiety, intraspecies aggression
    CAT: 10–20 mg/kg SC/IM

Megestrol acetate (Ovaban, Megace)
Lymphoplasmacytic stomatitis, eosinophilic granuloma
    Chapter 27
    CAT: 0.25 mg/kg PO QOD × 3 doses, then 1–2 times/wk
Prostatic hyperplasia (not approved for this use)
    Chapter 52
    DOG: 0.55 mg/kg PO SID × 4 wk
Galactorrhea
    Chapter 59
    DOG: 2 mg/kg PO SID × 5 days
Refractory eosinophilic keratitis and conjunctivitis
    Chapters 94, 96
    CAT: 0.5 mg/kg/day PO × 7–14 days; use with caution

Meglumine antimonate
Leishmaniasis
    Chapters 84, 114
    DOG: 100–200 mg/kg IV/SC SID–QOD × 3–4 wk

Melarsomine (Immiticide)
Heartworm adulticide
    Chapter 12
    DOG: a) 2.5 mg/kg IM SID × 2 days
        b) 2.5 mg/kg IM, wait 30 days, then give 2 more doses 24 hr apart

Melatonin
Canine pattern or flank alopecia
    Chapter 83
    DOG: 3–6 mg PO BID–TID × 4–6 wk
Alopecia X
    Chapter 88
    DOG: 3–6 mg PO BID–TID

Melphalan (Alkeran)
Thrombocythemia
Chapter 65
CAT: 0.5 mg PO SID × 4 days, then QOD
Multiple myeloma
Chapters 70, 75
DOG: a) 0.1 mg/kg PO/IV SID × 10 days, then 0.05 mg/kg PO SID × 2 wk, then 0.05 mg/kg PO QOD
b) 7 mg/m^2 PO SID × 5 days q 3 wk
c) 1.5 mg/m^2 PO SID × 7–10 days; repeat every 3 wk

Meperidine HCl (Demerol)
Analgesia
Chapters 35, 135
DOG: 3–10 mg/kg IM PRN or 2–4 mg/kg IV q 2 h
CAT: 2–4 mg/kg IM/SC PRN
Sedation, pain control
Chapter 122
DOG: 5–10 mg/kg IM
CAT: 1–4 mg/kg IM

2-Mercaptopropionyl glycine, Tiopronin (Thiola)
Cystine urolithiasis
Chapter 49
DOG: 15–25 mg/kg PO BID

6-Mercaptopurine (Purinethol)
Chronic myelocytic leukemia, lymphoma
DOG: 50 mg/m^2 PO SID or 2 mg/kg PO SID, in a protocol

Methazolamide (Neptazane)
Glaucoma
Chapter 98
DOG: 2–4 mg/kg PO BID–TID
CAT: 1–2 mg/kg PO BID

Methimazole (Tapazole)
Hyperthyroidism
> Chapter 41
> **CAT: a)** 2.5–5 mg PO BID
>   **b)** 1.25–2.5 mg PO BID if renal insufficiency present

Methocarbamol (Robaxin)
Muscle relaxation for intervertebral disk disease
> **DOG:** 15–20 mg/kg PO TID

**Muscle relaxation for certain toxicoses,
heat prostration**
> Chapters 122–129, 134
> **DOG:** 10% soln: 50–150 mg/kg IV; max = 300 mg/kg/day

Methoprene (Frontline Plus)
Flea growth inhibitor
> Chapter 87
> Apply topically once monthly, as directed

Methotrexate Na (Methotrexate)
Chemotherapy
> Chapters 67, 70
> **DOG:** 2.5 mg/m^2 PO SID–BID or 0.6–0.8 mg/kg IV q 3 wk,
>   in a protocol
> **CAT:** 0.8 mg/kg IV/PO q 4 wk

Methoxamine HCl (Vasoxyl)
Vasopressor: cardiac arrest, shock
> **DOG:** 0.1–0.8 mg/kg IV slowly

Methylphenidate (Ritalin)
Narcolepsy
> Chapter 22
> **DOG:** 0.25 mg/kg PO SID–BID

Methylprednisolone (Medrol)
Inflammatory bowel disease
> Chapter 32
> **CAT:** 1 mg/kg PO BID

Methylprednisolone acetate (Depo-Medrol)
Feline allergic bronchitis
Chapter 17
CAT: 10–20 mg IM q 2–8 wk
Eosinophilic ulcers and linear granulomas, lymphoplasmacytic stomatitis
Chapters 27, 85, 86
CAT: 2–4 mg/kg or 20–40 mg SC/IM q 2–6 wk × 2–6 Rx
Hypoadrenocorticism
Chapter 44
CAT: 10 mg IM q 3–4 wk
Tenosynovitis of biceps tendon
Chapter 80
DOG: 10–40 mg intrasynovially q 2 wk × 2 Rx
Allergic skin disease
Chapter 89
CAT: 20 mg SC/IM
Fibrous histiocytoma
Chapter 91
DOG: 10–40 mg sublesionally
Pannus, episcleritis, anterior uveitis
Chapters 96, 97
DOG: 4–8 mg subconjunctivally

Methylprednisolone sodium succinate (Solu-Medrol)
Cerebral and spinal trauma, fibrocartilaginous emboli
Chapters 23, 24
30 mg/kg IV, then 15 mg/kg IV 2 and 6 hr later, then
15 mg/kg IV QID × 2 days

4-Methylpyrazole (Antizol-Vet)
Ethylene glycol toxicosis
Chapters 122, 127
DOG: 20 mg/kg IV, then 15 mg/kg IV at 12 and 24 hr, then
5 mg/kg IV at 36 hr

Methyltestosterone (Estratest, Android)
Galactorrhea
> Chapter 59
> **DOG:** 1–2 mg/kg PO SID × 5–7 days; max = 25 mg/day

Testosterone-responsive dermatosis, alopecia X
> Chapter 88
> **DOG:** 0.5–1 mg/kg PO QOD; max = 30 mg/day

Metipranolol 0.3% (OptiPranolol)
Nonselective β-blocker for glaucoma
> Apply 1 drop to affected eye BID

Metoclopramide (Reglan)
Gastric motility disorders, antiemetic
> Chapters 29–35, 37, 110
> **DOG:** 0.2–0.5 mg/kg PO/SC TID–QID or
> 0.01–0.08 mg/kg/hr IV infusion
> **CAT:** 0.1–0.2 mg/kg PO TID or 0.01 mg/kg/hr IV as CRI

Gastric reflux
> Chapters 15, 17, 29, 128
> **DOG:** 0.2–0.4 mg/kg PO TID–QID

Dysautonomia
> **CAT:** 0.3 mg/kg PO TID

Metronidazole (Flagyl)
Hepatic encephalopathy
> Chapter 23
> **DOG:** 7.5 mg/kg PO TID

Meningitis
> Chapter 24
> **DOG:** 10–20 mg/kg PO TID

Stomatitis
> Chapter 27
> 15 mg/kg PO BID–TID, then taper to SID

Helicobacter
> Chapters 30, 111
> **DOG:** 15 mg/kg PO TID
> **CAT:** 62.5 mg/day PO SID

GI tract bacterial overgrowth, acute colitis, perianal fistulas
Chapters 32–37
DOG: 7.5–15 mg/kg PO BID–TID or 10 mg/kg IV over
30 min
CAT: 10 mg/kg/day PO
EPI
Chapter 35
DOG: 7.5 mg/kg PO BID–TID
CAT: 20–100 mg PO BID × 14 days
Giardia, Entamoeba, Trichomonas, Balantidium, Babesia
Chapters 32, 33, 114
DOG: 10–30 mg/kg PO SID–BID × 5–7 days
CAT: 10–25 mg/kg PO SID–BID × 5 days
Osteomyelitis, cellulitis
Chapters 79, 84
15 mg/kg IV or 25 mg/kg PO BID

Mexiletine (Mexitil)
Ventricular arrhythmia
Chapters 7, 31
DOG: 4–8 mg/kg PO TID

Mibolerone (Cheque)
Galactorrhea
Chapter 59
DOG: 16 µg/kg PO SID × 5 days
Prevent estrus (dogs only)
1–11 kg: 30 µg/day PO
12–22 kg: 60 µg/day PO
23–45 kg: 120 µg/day PO
>45 kg: 180 µg/day PO
**German shepherd dog, German shepherd dog
cross:** 180 µg/day PO

Miconazole (Conofite, Monistat IV)
Dermatophytosis (Conofite)
Apply topically as directed

Miconazole (Conofite, Monistat IV) *(continued)*
Ocular fungal infections (Monistat IV)
Chapter 96
Apply topically 4–12 times daily

Midazolam (Versed)
Preanesthetic, sedation
Chapter 31
DOG: 0.1–0.2 mg/kg IM/SC/IV

Milbemycin oxime (Interceptor)
Heartworm prophylaxis, hookworm and whipworm prophylaxis, microfilaricide
Chapters 12, 32, 33
0.5 mg/kg PO monthly
Pneumonyssoides **infection**
Chapter 14
0.5–1.0 mg/kg PO once weekly × 3 wk
Demodicosis in adult dogs
Chapters 87, 93
DOG: 2 mg/kg PO SID × 60–90 days PRN
Sarcoptic mange
Chapter 87
DOG: 2 mg/kg PO once or twice weekly × 3 wk

Minocycline (Minocin)
Brucellosis, diskospondylitis
Chapters 24, 111
DOG: 12.5 mg/kg PO BID with gentamicin
Rickettsial infections
Chapter 113
DOG: 10 mg/kg PO/IV BID × 10 days

Misoprostol (Cytotec)
Unresponsive atopy, pruritus
Chapter 89
DOG: 6 µg/kg PO TID
Gastrointestinal protectant
Chapters 30, 128
DOG: 3–5 µg/kg PO TID–QID

Mithramycin (Mithracin)
Hypercalcemia
> Chapter 71
> > 0.1–0.2 µg/kg IV SID × 2 Rx

Mitotane (Lysodren)
Pituitary-dependent hyperadrenocorticism
> Chapters 44, 88
> > **DOG:** 25–50 mg/kg/day PO SID × 5–10 days, then
> > q 4–7 days or PRN

Functional adrenocortical tumors
> Chapter 70
> > **DOG:** 50–75 mg/kg PO dd BID initially, then
> > 50–100 mg/kg/wk PO

Mitoxantrone (Novantrone)
Chemotherapy, in a protocol
> Chapters 41, 70
> > **DOG:** 5.5–6 mg/m^2 IV q 3 wk
> > **CAT:** 5–6.5 mg/m^2 IV q 3 wk

Modafinil (Profigil)
Narcolepsy
> Chapter 22
> > **DOG:** 1–5 mg/kg/day PO

Morphine SO$_4$ (Duramorph)
Supraventricular premature beats
> Chapters 8, 9
> > **DOG:** 0.1–0.2 mg/kg IM/IV/SC PRN

Analgesia
> Chapters 31, 37, 79, 105, 132, 133, 135
> > **DOG:** 0.2–0.5 mg/kg SC/IM q 4–6 h or 0.1 mg/kg IV
> > BID–QID
> > **CAT:** 0.05–0.1 mg/kg SC/IM BID

Spinal trauma
> Chapter 24
> > **DOG:** 0.5–1.0 mg/kg IM/SC q 4–6 h

Moxidectin (ProHeart-6)
Heartworm prophylaxis
  Chapter 12
  DOG: 0.17 mg/kg SC every 6 mo

Naloxone HCl (Narcan)
Stereotypic behavior
  DOG: 20 mg SC
Narcotic antagonist
  Chapter 122
  0.02–0.04 mg/kg IV

Naltrexone (Trexan)
Acral lick granuloma
  Chapter 86
  DOG: 2.2 mg/kg PO SID–BID
  CAT: 2.2 mg/kg PO SID

Nandrolone decanoate (Deca-Durabolin)
Thrombocythemia
  Chapter 65
  CAT: 15 mg IM once
Anabolic effects, myelofibrosis
  Chapters 65, 71
  DOG: 1–5 mg/kg/wk IM; max = 200 mg
  CAT: 10–20 mg/wk IM

Natamycin 5% (Pimaricin)
Ocular fungal infections
  Chapter 96
  Apply topically 3–8 times daily

Neostigmine (Prostigmin)
Myasthenia gravis
  Chapter 25
  DOG: 0.05 mg/kg IM TID–QID

Niacinamide (Glutofac)
Metatarsal fistulation, sterile pyogranulomas
>Chapters 82, 85
>**DOG:** 250–500 mg PO BID–TID, with tetracycline

Pemphigus, discoid lupus, episcleritis
>Chapters 89, 96
>**DOG:** 250–500 mg PO TID, with tetracycline

Nicotinamide (niacin, nicotinic acid)
Vacor toxicosis
>Chapters 122, 123
>50–100 mg IM × 2 wk

Nifurtimox (Lampit) (not available in USA)
Trypanosomiasis
>**DOG:** 2 mg/kg PO QID × 3 mo

Nitenpyran (Capstar)
Flea adulticide
>Chapter 87
>**DOG OR CAT:** 2–25 lbs: 11.4 mg
>**DOG:** 25–125 lbs: 57.0 mg

Nitroglycerin 2% ointment (Nitro-Bid, Nitrol)
Dilatative cardiomyopathy, heart failure
>Chapter 9
>**DOG:** 0.25–1 in. cutaneously q 4–6 h
>**CAT:** 1/8–1/4 in. cutaneously QID

Nitroprusside (Nipride, Nitropress)
Vasodilator for acute congestive heart failure
>Chapter 9
>**DOG:** 1–10 µg/kg/min IV infusion

Nizatidine (Axid)
Constipation, megacolon
>Chapter 33
>**CAT:** 2.5–5 mg/kg PO SID

Nizatidine (Axid) *(continued)*
Gastric ulcers
>**DOG:** 5 mg/kg PO SID

Nystatin (Mycolog, Nilstat)
Candidiasis
>Apply topically BID–TID × 1–2 wk

Octreotide acetate (Sandostatin)
Glucagonoma, gastrinoma
>Chapter 43
>**DOG:** 10–40 µg/kg SC BID–TID

Omeprazole (Prilosec)
Reflux esophagitis, GI ulceration
>Chapters 29, 30, 32, 37
>**DOG:** 0.5–1.0 mg/kg PO SID, max = 20 mg

Ondansetron (Zofran ODT)
Antiemetic
>Chapters 32, 37
>**DOG:** 0.1–0.2 mg/kg SC TID

o,p′-DDD
>*See* Mitotane

Ormetoprim/sulfa (Primor)
>*See* Sulfadimethoxine/ormetoprim

Oxacillin (Bactocill, Prostaphilin)
Staphylococcus infections
>Chapters 79, 84
>20 mg/kg PO/IV/IM TID–QID

Oxazepam (Serax)
Appetite stimulant
>Chapter 109
>**CAT:** 2–3 mg PO SID–BID

Oxybutynin (Ditropan)
Detrusor hyperspasticity
Chapter 50
DOG: 0.2 mg/kg PO BID–TID or 1.25–5 mg PO BID–TID in large dogs
CAT: 0.5–1.25 mg PO BID–TID

Oxyglobin, purified bovine hemoglobin (Oxyglo$_2$bin)
Hypoxia in acute abdomen syndrome
Chapter 37
DOG: 5 ml/kg IV
Red blood cell substitute
Chapter 69
DOG: 10–30 ml/kg IV at 10 ml/kg/hr CRI

Oxymetholone (Anadrol-50)
Anabolic agent
Chapter 63
1 mg/kg PO SID–BID

Oxymorphone (Numorphan)
Sedation
Chapters 15, 17
DOG: 0.05–0.1 mg/kg IV or 0.1–0.2 mg/kg IM/SC
CAT: 0.02 mg/kg IV
Analgesia
Chapters 8, 24, 31, 79, 133, 135
DOG: 0.025–0.2 mg/kg IV/IM/SC q 4–6 h
CAT: 0.025–0.05 mg/kg IV/SC q 4–6 h
Preanesthetic, during gastric dilatation
Chapter 31
DOG: 0.1–0.2 mg/kg IV; max = 3 mg

Oxytetracycline (Urobiotic-250, Terramycin)
Hemobartonellosis, EPI, *Mycoplasma*
Chapters 35, 112, 113
DOG: 20–40 mg/kg PO TID × 3 wk
CAT: 15–30 mg/kg PO BID–TID × 3 wk or 50–100 mg PO BID

Oxytocin (Pitocin, Syntocinon)
Uterine prolapse
Chapter 56
DOG: 5–10 U IM/SC once
Stimulate milk letdown
Chapter 59
DOG: a) Spray intranasally in the bitch 5–10 min before nursing
b) 2–20 IU SC/IM
CAT: 1–10 IU SC/IM
Uterine inertia
Chapters 60, 61
DOG: a) 2–10 U IM or IV infusion; may repeat in 30–60 min
b) 10 U in 5% D/W IV over 30 min
CAT: 1–3 U IM/SC; may repeat in 20–30 min

Pamidronate (Aredia)
Hypercalcemia
Chapter 42
DOG: 1.3 mg/kg in 0.9% NaCl IV over 2–4 hr

Pancreatic enzymes (Viokase, Pancreazyme)
Pancreatic exocrine insufficiency
Chapter 35
DOG: 1–2 tsp/20 kg with each meal until normal, then taper
CAT: 0.5 tsp/5 kg with food until normal, then taper

Pancuronium bromide (Pavulon)
Paralytic agent
Chapter 134
DOG: 0.04–0.1 mg/kg IV initially, then
0.06–0.1 mg/kg/hr IV

Paromomycin (Humatin)
Cryptosporidiosis, trichomoniasis
Chapters 32, 114
DOG: 125–165 mg/kg PO BID × 5 days

■ **Paroxetine (Paxil)**
Certain behavioral disorders
> Chapter 117
> **CAT:** 0.5 mg/kg PO SID–BID

■ **D-Penicillamine (Cuprimine)**
Copper hepatopathy
> Chapter 34
> **DOG:** 10–15 mg/kg/day PO
Cystine urolithiasis
> Chapter 49
> **DOG:** 15 mg/kg PO BID with food
Lead and zinc poisoning
> Chapters 122, 127
> **DOG:** 35–50 mg/kg/day PO dd QID × 7 days; wait 7 days,
> then repeat

■ **Penicillin, aqueous (K or Na)**
Meningitis, bacterial endocarditis
> Chapters 9, 24
> 20,000–50,000 U/kg IV q 4–6 h
Actinomycosis, tetanus
> Chapters 111, 126
> **a)** 22,000 U/kg IV QID or 1,000,000 U intralesionally
> **b)** 40 mg/kg PO TID

■ **Penicillin, procaine (Wycillin)**
Leptospirosis, actinomycosis
> Chapter 47
> 20,000–50,000 U/kg IM/SC BID

■ **Pentamidine (phenamidine) isethionate (Pentam)**
Babesiosis
> **DOG:** 15 mg/kg SC SID × 2 days

Pentobarbital (Nembutal)
Status epilepticus, strychnine and other toxicities
Chapters 22, 122, 123, 126
2–15 mg/kg IV or 5 mg/kg/hr IV to effect
Sedation
Chapter 134
0.2–1 mg/kg/hr IV
Anesthesia
10–30 mg/kg IV to effect

Pentoxifylline (Trental)
Dermatomyositis, contact dermatitis
Chapters 82, 89
DOG: 10 mg/kg PO BID–TID, with food
Cutaneous vasculitis
Chapter 89
DOG: 10–15 mg/kg PO QOD
Pneumocystis carinii
DOG: 4 mg/kg IM/SC × 2 wk

Phenobarbital
Antitussive
DOG: 2 mg/kg PO at bedtime
Seizures
Chapters 22, 23, 110
DOG: 1–2.5 mg/kg PO BID initially; some require up to
20 mg/kg/day
CAT: 2.5 mg/kg PO SID
Status epilepticus
Chapters 22, 122
a) 2–4 mg/kg IV repeated to effect; max = 20 mg/kg or
≤100 mg/min IV until serum level = 25 µg/ml (dogs) or
15 µg/ml (cats)
b) 2–10 mg/kg IM
Sedation
DOG: 1–2 mg/kg PO BID–TID
CAT: 1 mg/kg PO BID
Acral lick dermatitis, psychogenic alopecia
Chapter 86
2–6 mg/kg PO BID

Phenoxybenzamine HCl (Dibenzyline)
Acute hypertension from pheochromocytoma
Chapter 44
DOG: 0.2–1.5 mg/kg PO BID
Functional urethral obstruction
Chapter 50
DOG: 0.25 mg/kg PO BID
CAT: 1.25–7.5 mg PO SID–BID

Phenylbutazone (Butazolidin)
Anti-inflammatory, arthritis
Chapter 78
8–10 mg/kg PO TID × 48 hr, then taper to lowest
effective dose; max = 800 mg/day

Phenylephrine (Neo-Synephrine)
Vasopressor
Chapters 122, 128
DOG: 0.15 mg/kg IV

Phenylpropanolamine HCl
Urethral sphincter incompetence
Chapters 50, 116
DOG: 12.5–50 mg PO BID–TID or 1.5 mg/kg PO BID–TID
CAT: 1.5–2.2 mg/kg PO BID–TID

Phenytoin (Dilantin)
Ventricular arrhythmias
Chapter 122
DOG: 2–4 mg/kg IV in increments; max = 10 mg/kg

Physostigmine (Antilirium)
Muscarinic mushroom intoxication
Chapter 129
DOG: 0.02 mg/kg IM

Physostigmine 0.25% ophthalmic ointment (Eserine)
Dysautonomia
> Chapter 103
> **CAT:** Apply ⅛ in. topically BID–TID

Phytomenadione
> *See* Vitamin K₁

Pilocarpine 1–2% ophthalmic solution
KCS
> Chapter 95
> **DOG:** 1–4 drops on food BID–TID
Dysautonomia
> Chapter 103
> **CAT:** 1 drop topically QID
Glaucoma
> Chapters 98, 99
> 1 drop to affected eye BID–QID

Piroxicam (Feldene)
Transitional cell carcinoma, analgesia for cancer-induced pain
> Chapters 49, 51, 52, 70, 95
> **DOG:** 0.3 mg/kg PO SID
> **CAT:** 0.3 mg/kg PO QOD, with misoprostol

Pitressin tannate
Diabetes insipidus
> Chapter 40
> **DOG:** 2.5–5 U IM q 24–72 h

Plasma, fresh frozen
Hypoproteinemia
> Chapters 32, 69
> 10–20 ml/kg IV
Pancreatitis
> Chapter 35
> **DOG:** 50–250 ml IV SID

Von Willebrand's disease, clotting factor deficiencies
    Chapters 66, 69
    6–20 mg/kg IV
Burns
    Chapter 133
    0.5 ml/kg × % body surface area burned
DIC
    Chapters 69, 134
    5–10 ml/kg IV

■ Plicamycin
    See Mithramycin

■ Polysulfated glycosaminoglycans (Adequan)
DJD
    Chapter 78
    DOG: 5 mg/kg IM once weekly × 6–8 wk

■ Potassium bromide
Seizures
    Chapters 22, 23
    DOG: 20–40 mg/kg PO SID or divided BID with food
    CAT: 30 mg/kg PO SID

■ Potassium chloride, injectable
Serum potassium deficit
    Chapters 31, 32, 43
    a) 2–10 mEq/kg/day added to IV fluids
    b) 20–40 mEq added to each liter IV fluids
Hypokalemic polymyopathy
    Chapter 80
    0.4 mEq/kg/hr as 40–80 mEq KCl per liter IV fluids

■ Potassium citrate (Citrolith)
Chronic renal failure
    Chapter 47
    30 mg/kg PO BID

Potassium citrate (Citrolith) *(continued)*
Urine alkalization
    Chapter 49
    40–75 mg/kg PO BID

Potassium gluconate (Tumil-K)
Hypokalemia, hypokalemic polymyopathy
    Chapters 47, 80, 120
    CAT: 2–6 mEq PO SID–BID

Potassium iodide (SSKI Solution)
Sporotrichosis
    Chapter 84
    DOG: 40 mg/kg PO BID–TID
    CAT: 10–20 mg/kg PO SID–TID

Potassium permanganate (1:2000)
Strychnine and nicotine toxicosis
    Chapters 122, 123, 128, 129
    5 ml/kg in gastric lavage

Potassium phosphate
Serum phosphate deficit
    Chapter 43
    0.03 mmol/kg/hr IV

Pralidoxime Cl (2PAM, Protopam)
Organophosphate toxicosis
    Chapters 122, 124
    20 mg/kg IV BID

Praziquantel (Droncit, Drontal Plus)
Tapeworms: *Taenia, Dipylidium*
    Chapter 32
    DOG: 0.5 tab/2.5 kg PO; max = 5 tab
    CAT: 1.8 kg: 0.5 tab PO
         2.3–5 kg: 1 tab PO
         >5 kg: 1.5 tab PO

Pancreatic flukes
> Chapter 35
> **CAT:** 40 mg/kg PO SID × 3 days

Nanophyetus salminocola
> Chapter 113
> **DOG:** 10–30 mg/kg PO/SC once

▪ Prazosin (Minipress)

Systemic hypertension
> Chapter 47
> **DOG:** 1 mg/10–15 kg PO SID–TID

Decrease urethral resistance
> Chapter 50
> **DOG:** 1 mg PO SID–BID
> **CAT:** 0.25–0.5 mg PO SID–BID or 0.03 mg/kg IV

▪ Prednisolone, prednisone (Deltasone)

Allergic bronchitis, asthma, heartworm disease
> Chapters 12, 17
> 0.5–2 mg/kg IM/PO BID

Chronic bronchitis, tracheitis, laryngitis
> Chapters 15–17
> **DOG:** 0.1–0.2 mg/kg PO BID

Pulmonary eosinophilic infiltrates
> Chapter 18
> 0.5–2 mg/kg PO BID

Acquired tremors
> Chapter 23
> **DOG:** 1–2 mg/kg PO BID

Hydrocephalus, syringomyelia
> Chapter 23, 24
> **DOG:** 0.25–0.5 mg/kg PO BID–QOD

Cerebral edema from brain or spinal tumors
> Chapters 23, 24
> 0.5–1 mg/kg PO SID–BID, taper to QOD

Idiopathic/eosinophilic meningitis, granulomatous meningoencephalitis
> Chapter 23
> **DOG:** 1–2 mg/kg IM/PO BID, then taper

Prednisolone, prednisone (Deltasone) *(continued)*
Meningitis–arteritis
  Chapter 24
  DOG: 4 mg/kg/day PO × 7–14 days, then taper to
     0.5 mg/kg PO QOD × 6 mo
**Intervertebral disk disease, spondylopathy, cauda
equina syndrome**
  Chapter 24
  DOG: 0.5 mg/kg PO SID
Acquired myasthenia gravis
  Chapter 25
  DOG: 0.25 mg/kg PO initially; slowly increase to
     2 mg/kg/day PO until remission, then taper to QOD
**Relapsing or chronic inflammatory demyelinating
neuropathy**
  Chapter 25
  1–2 mg/kg PO BID
Eosinophilic ulcers, lymphoplasmacytic gingivitis
  Chapters 27, 85
  DOG: 1–2.2 mg/kg PO SID × 7 days, then taper dose to
     QOD
  CAT: 1–4 mg/kg PO BID
Plasmacytic/lymphocytic gastritis, enteritis
  Chapters 30, 32
  DOG: 1–2 mg/kg PO BID, taper dose weekly
  CAT: 2–4 mg/kg/day PO, then taper
Eosinophilic gastritis, enteritis, colitis
  Chapters 32, 33
  1–3 mg/kg PO SID–BID, taper to QOD
**Lymphocytic cholangitis, chronic active hepatitis,
copper hepatopathy**
  Chapter 34
  1 mg/kg PO BID, then taper
Perianal fistulas
  Chapter 36
  DOG: 2 mg/kg PO SID × 14 days, then taper
Hypercalcemia
  Chapters 42, 71, 123
  a) 1–3 mg/kg PO/SC SID–BID
  b) 40 mg/m^2 PO BID

Hypoadrenocorticism, hypopituitarism
>Chapters 40, 44
>0.2–0.4 mg/kg PO SID–QOD

Hypoglycemia
>Chapters 45, 71
>0.25–2 mg/kg PO SID–BID

Urethritis, persistent hematuria
>Chapters 49, 51
>1 mg/kg PO SID–BID × 14 days, then taper

Immune hemolytic anemia, myelodysplastic syndrome
>Chapters 63, 65
>1–2 mg/kg/day PO dd BID

Mast cell tumors, mastocytosis
>Chapters 70, 71, 91
>**DOG:** 30–40 mg/m² PO SID × 4 wk, then QOD, or
>>1–2 mg/kg PO SID–BID
>**CAT:** 40 mg/m² PO SID × 1 wk, then 20 mg/m² PO QOD

Immune thrombocytopenia
>Chapter 66
>2–3 mg/kg/day PO/IM dd BID, taper to 0.5–1 mg/kg PO
>>q 2–3 d

Lymphosarcoma, myeloproliferative disorders, eosinophilic leukemia
>Chapters 64, 67, 70
>a) 1–2 mg/kg PO SID, in a protocol
>b) 30–40 mg/m² PO SID × 2–4 wk, then QOD, in a protocol

Angioneurotic edema, urticaria
>Chapter 74
>1–2 mg/kg PO/IM SID–BID

Immune skin diseases, SLE
>Chapters 74, 89, 93
>1–2 mg/kg PO BID until remission, then taper

Cutaneous histiocytosis, fibrous histiocytoma
>Chapters 75, 91
>**DOG:** 1–2 mg/kg PO BID

Multiple myeloma, macroglobulinemia
>Chapter 75
>0.5 mg/kg PO SID, in a protocol

Prednisolone, prednisone (Deltasone) *(continued)*
SLE or rheumatoid arthritis
>   Chapter 78
>   1–2 mg/kg PO SID–BID, taper to ≤1 mg/kg PO QOD

Panosteitis, hypertrophic osteopathy
>   Chapter 79
>   **DOG:** 0.25–0.5 mg/kg PO SID

Immune polymyositis, masticatory myositis, dermatomyositis
>   Chapters 80, 82, 101
>   1–2 mg/kg PO/IM SID–BID × 3–4 wk, then taper

Canine atopy, contact allergy, flea allergy, acanthosis nigricans, vasculitis
>   Chapters 82, 84, 89
>   **DOG:** 0.5 mg/kg PO BID × 5–10 days, then taper
>   **CAT:** 1–2 mg/kg PO SID × 5–10 days, then taper

Sterile pyogranulomas, panniculitis
>   Chapter 85
>   **DOG:** 2–4 mg/kg/day PO
>   **CAT:** 4 mg/kg PO SID

Juvenile cellulitis, sebaceous adenitis
>   Chapter 85
>   **DOG:** 2.2 mg/kg PO SID

Food allergy, parasite hypersensitivity
>   Chapter 89
>   0.5 mg/kg PO SID–BID, taper weekly

Blepharitis, episcleritis, uveitis, chorioretinitis, ligneous conjunctivitis, optic neuritis
>   Chapters 93, 94, 96, 97, 100
>   0.5–2 mg/kg PO BID, then taper

Otitis externa, media
>   Chapters 105, 106
>   0.5–2.2 mg/kg/day PO, taper over 7–21 days

FIP
>   Chapter 110
>   **CAT:** 2–4 mg/kg PO SID–BID, with cyclophosphamide

Prednisolone acetate 1% (Econopred)
Anterior uveitis, pannus
    Chapters 96, 97, 99, 101
    Apply 1 drop to affected eye 2–12 times daily

Prednisolone sodium succinate (Solu-Delta-Cortef)
Shock, CPR, anaphylaxis
    Chapters 8, 31, 44, 74
    11–30 mg/kg IV
Feline allergic bronchitis, asthma
    Chapter 17
    CAT: 10–20 mg/kg IV/IM
Hypoglycemia
    1–2 mg/kg IV

Primaquine PO_4 (Primaquine) (not available in USA)
Babesiosis
    CAT: 0.5 mg/kg PO/IM/SC once

Procainamide (Procainamide, Procan SR)
Ventricular arrhythmias
    Chapters 7, 8, 10, 31
    DOG: a) 10–20 mg/kg IM/PO TID–QID
          b) 6–20 mg/kg IV slowly
          c) 25–50 µg/kg/min or to effect IV in 5% D/W
    CAT: a) 3–8 mg/kg PO TID–QID
          b) 1–2 mg/kg IV bolus
          c) 10–20 µg/kg/min IV in 5% D/W as CRI

Prochlorperazine (Compazine)
Antiemetic
    Chapters 32, 37, 110
    DOG: 0.05–0.5 mg/kg IM/SC BID–TID
    CAT: 0.125 mg/kg IM BID

Progesterone in oil
Hypoluteoidism
Chapter 60
DOG: 2 mg/kg IM q 3 days

Proligestone (Delvosteron) (not available in USA)
Galactorrhea
Chapter 59
DOG: 20–30 mg/kg SC

Promethazine (Phenergan)
Antihistamine, urticaria
0.2–0.4 mg/kg PO TID–QID

Propantheline bromide (Propantheline)
Sinus bradycardia
Chapter 7
0.25–0.5 mg/kg PO BID–TID
Irritable colon syndrome
Chapter 33
DOG: 0.25 mg/kg PO BID–TID
Decrease bladder contractility
Chapter 50
DOG: 7.5–15 mg PO BID–TID
CAT: 5–7.5 mg PO QOD–TID

Propofol (Rapinovet, Diprivan)
Status epilepticus
Chapter 22
DOG: 4–8 mg/kg IV to effect or 8–12 µg/kg/hr IV as CRI
Seizures associated with liver disease
Chapter 34
DOG: 1 mg/kg IV bolus, then 0.1–0.25 mg/kg/min IV as CRI

Anesthesia
> **CAT:** Induction: 7 mg/kg IV
> Maintenance: 0.51 mg/kg/min IV
> **DOG:** Induction: 2.5–3 mg/kg IV, with premedication

■ Propranolol (Inderal)

Ventricular arrhythmias
> Chapters 7, 9
> **DOG:** 0.01–0.10 mg/kg IV over 10 min or 0.2–1 mg/kg PO
> BID–TID; max = 1 mg/kg/day PO

Tachyarrhythmias from endocrinopathies, certain toxicoses
> Chapters 7, 41, 44, 129
> **DOG:** 0.15–1.0 mg/kg PO TID or 0.01–0.1 mg/kg IV over
> 5–10 min
> **CAT:** 2.5–5 mg PO BID–TID

Acquired tremors
> Chapter 23
> **DOG:** 1 mg/kg PO TID

Hypertrophic cardiomyopathy
> **CAT:** ≤4.5 kg: 2.5 mg PO BID–TID
> **CAT:** ≥5 kg: 5 mg PO BID–TID

Hypertension
> Chapters 44, 47
> **DOG:** 2.5–80 mg or 0.15 mg/kg PO BID–TID
> **CAT:** 2.5–10 mg PO BID–TID

Hypoglycemia
> Chapter 71
> **DOG:** 10–40 mg PO TID

Certain behavioral disorders
> Chapter 116
> **DOG:** 5–10 mg PO BID–TID

■ Prostaglandin $F_{2\alpha}$ (Lutalyse)

Pyometritis, open
> Chapters 56, 60, 61
> **DOG:** 0.1–0.25 mg/kg SC SID–BID × 5–7 days
> **CAT:** 0.1–0.25 mg/kg SC SID–TID

Protamine sulfate (Protamine)
Antagonist to heparin
   Chapter 18
   DOG: 1 mg per 100 U heparin to be inactivated

Pseudoephedrine (Actifed, Sudafed)
Rhinitis
   Chapter 14
   DOG: 15–50 mg PO BID–TID; max = 4 mg/kg
   CAT: 2–4 mg/kg PO BID–TID
Retrograde ejaculation
   Chapter 60
   DOG: 4–5 mg/kg PO, 1 and 3 hr before breeding

Psyllium (Metamucil, Alarmucil)
Bulk laxative
   DOG: 2–4 tsp PO PRN in food
   CAT: 1–2 tsp PO SID–BID in food

Pyrantel pamoate (Nemex, Strongid-T)
Roundworms, hookworms
   Chapter 32
   5–10 mg/kg (1 ml/5–10 lbs) PO; repeat in 3 wk

Pyridostigmine bromide (Mestinon)
Myasthenia gravis
   Chapter 25
   DOG: 0.2 2 mg/kg PO BID–TID

Pyridoxine HCl (vitamin B_6)
Crimidine and ethylene glycol toxicosis
   Chapters 123, 127
   DOG: 20 mg/kg IV

Pyrimethamine (Daraprim)
Toxoplasmosis, neosporosis, hepatozoonosis
> Chapters 25, 80, 100, 114
> > **DOG:** 0.25–0.5 mg/kg PO SID–BID × 2–4 wk, with
> > sulfonamides

Pyriproxifen (Indorex)
Flea growth inhibitor
> Chapter 87
> Apply topically once monthly, as directed

Quinacrine (Atabrine)
Giardia
> 9–11 mg/kg PO SID × 6–12 days

Quinidine, Q. gluconate (Quinaglute), Q. polygalacturonate (Cardioquin), Q. sulfate (Quinidex)
Ventricular arrhythmias
> Chapter 7
> 6–20 mg/kg IM/PO TID–QID

Ranitidine HCl (Zantac)
Esophagitis, gastric reflux, megacolon
> Chapters 29, 33
> > **DOG:** 2 mg/kg PO BID–TID
> > **CAT:** 1–2 mg/kg PO BID

Chronic gastritis, GI tract ulceration, EPI, enteric viruses
> Chapters 15, 17, 30–32, 35, 37, 71, 110, 128
> > **DOG:** 0.5–2.0 mg/kg IV/SC/PO BID–TID
> > **CAT:** 0.5 mg/kg IV BID or 2.5 mg/kg PO BID

Hypergastrinemia from chronic renal failure
> Chapter 47
> > **DOG:** 1–2 mg/kg PO BID or 0.5 mg/kg IV/SC BID

Effects of mast cell tumors
> Chapter 91
> 0.5–2 mg/kg IV/PO BID

Rifampin (Rifamate, Rifadin)
Tuberculosis
>Chapter 111
>**DOG:** 10–20 mg/kg PO BID–TID
>**CAT:** 5 mg PO SID

Rutin
Lymphedema, chylothorax
>Chapters 19, 67
>**DOG:** 50 mg/kg PO TID

Safflower oil
Mycosis fungoides
>Chapter 91
>**DOG:** 3 ml/kg PO mixed with food twice weekly

SAMe (Denosyl)
Chronic hepatitis
>Chapter 34
>**DOG:** 18 mg/kg PO SID

Selamectin (Revolution)
Heartworm prophylaxis
>Chapter 12
>6 mg/kg PO once monthly
Sarcoptic, notoedric, and otodectic mange
>Chapters 87, 93
>6–12 mg/kg topically q 2–4 wk × 1–3 Rx
Ear mites
>Chapter 87
>1–2 applications, 4 weeks apart
Flea adulticide
>Chapter 87
>Apply topically once monthly, as directed

Selegiline
>*See* L-Deprenyl

Sertraline (Zoloft)
Certain behavioral disorders
Chapters 116, 117
DOG: 1 mg/kg PO SID
CAT: 0.5 mg/kg PO SID–BID

Sodium bicarbonate
CPR, atrial standstill
Chapters 7, 8
0.5–1 mEq/kg IV q 5–10 min
Severe acidemia
Chapter 31
1–2 mEq/kg IV
Hyperkalemia in acute renal failure
Chapter 47
0.5–2 mEq/kg IV over 20–30 min
Chronic renal failure
Chapter 47
15 mg/kg PO TID
Urine alkalization
Chapter 49
10–90 gr/day PO
Certain toxicoses
Chapters 122–129
50 mg/kg PO BID–TID

Sodium chloride (salt tablets)
Hypoadrenocorticism
1–5 g/day PO

Sodium chloride 5% ophthalmic ointment (Muro 128)
Corneal edema, nonhealing erosions
Chapter 96
Apply ⅛ in. topically 2–6 times daily

Sodium chloride 7.5%
See Hypertonic saline

Sodium iodide, 20% solution
Sporotrichosis
CAT: 0.5 ml/5 kg/day PO

Sodium phosphate (K-Phos)
Hypercalcemia
Dilute 1–3 g with water (1:1); give 10–20 ml PO
SID–TID until stools are soft

Sodium stibogluconate (Pentostam)
Leishmaniasis
Chapter 114
DOG: 30–50 mg/kg SC SID × 3–4 wk

Sodium sulfate (GoLYTELY)
Cathartic
Chapter 122
1 g/kg PO

Sodium thiopental (Pentothal)
Anesthesia
3–15 mg/kg IV to effect

Somatostatin
See Octreotide acetate

Sorbitol 70% (Actidose with Sorbitol)
Cathartic
Chapter 122
1–3 ml/kg PO

Sotalol (Betapace)
Atrial, ventricular tachycardia
Chapter 7
1–2 mg/kg PO BID

Spironolactone (Aldactone)
Diuretic: heart failure, hypertension
Chapters 9, 47
DOG: 1–2 mg/kg PO SID–BID
Primary hyperaldosteronism, noncirrhotic portal hypertension
Chapter 34
DOG: 1–2 mg/kg PO BID
CAT: 12.5 mg PO SID

Stanozolol (Winstrol)
Anabolic agent
Chapter 71
DOG: 1–4 mg PO BID
CAT: 1–2 mg PO BID

Stilbestrol
Hormone-responsive incontinence
Chapter 50
DOG: 0.04–0.06 mg PO SID × 1 wk, then taper to 0.01 mg/day

Streptomycin (Streptomycin)
Leptospirosis, endocarditis, tuberculosis
Chapters 18, 47
DOG: 10 mg/kg IM BID–QID
Brucellosis
Chapter 60
DOG: 20 mg/kg IM SID × 14 days

Succimer (Chemet)
Lead and arsenic poisoning
Chapters 122, 127
DOG: 10 mg/kg PO TID × 10 days

Sucralfate (Carafate)
Esophagitis, GI tract ulceration
> Chapters 29, 30, 32, 37, 44, 78, 128
> **DOG:** a) 0.5–1 g/25 kg PO BID–QID
> b) 0.5–1 g crushed and mixed with 10 ml water;
> give 5–10 ml slurry PO TID
> **CAT:** 250–500 mg PO BID–TID

Sulfadiazine (Sulfadiazine)
> *See also* Trimethoprim/sulfadiazine
Toxoplasmosis
> Chapters 25, 100
> 30–50 mg/kg PO BID × 14 days, with pyrimethamine

Sulfadimethoxine (Bactrovet, Albon)
Coccidiosis
> Chapters 32, 114
> 50 mg/kg PO SID once, then 25 mg/kg PO SID × 5–20 days

Sulfadimethoxine/Ormetoprim (Primor)
Bacterial folliculitis
> Chapter 84
> **DOG:** 27.5 mg/kg PO SID × 14 days
Coccidiosis
> Chapter 114
> **DOG:** 55 mg/kg PO SID × 7–23 days

Sulfasalazine (Azulfidine)
Chronic colitis
> Chapter 33
> **DOG:** 10–20 mg/kg PO TID; max = 3 g/day
> **CAT:** 10 mg/kg PO SID–BID; use with caution
Cutaneous vasculitis, subcorneal pustular dermatosis
> Chapters 85, 89
> **DOG:** 10–20 mg/kg PO TID until remission, then taper

Suprofen 1% (Profenal)
Anterior uveitis
Chapter 97
Apply 1 drop to affected eye BID–QID

Tamoxifen (Nolvadex)
Mammary neoplasia
DOG: 0.42 mg/kg/day PO

Taurine
Dilatative cardiomyopathy
Chapters 10, 120
DOG: 500 mg PO BID–TID
CAT: 250–500 mg PO BID
Central retinal degeneration
Chapters 100, 120
CAT: 250–500 mg PO SID–BID

Terbutaline (Brethine)
Bronchodilator
Chapters 16, 17, 132
DOG: a) 0.625–2.5 mg PO BID–TID
b) 0.03 mg/kg PO TID
c) 0.01 mg/kg IM/SC TID–QID
CAT: a) 0.625 mg PO BID
b) 0.01 mg/kg IM/SC

Terfenadine (Seldane)
Antihistamine, allergic skin disease
DOG: 2.5–5 mg/kg PO BID

Testosterone cypionate (Virilon)
Hormone-responsive incontinence
Chapter 50
DOG: 200 mg IM monthly

Testosterone, methyl

See Methyltestosterone

Testosterone propionate (in oil)

Hormone-responsive incontinence
    Chapter 50
    DOG: 2 mg/kg SC/IM 3 times/wk
    CAT: 5–10 mg IM PRN
Decrease milk production in pseudocyesis
    Chapter 60
    DOG: 0.5–1.0 mg/kg IM
Feline symmetrical alopecia
    Chapter 83
    CAT: 12.5 mg IM, with estrogen
Hormonal hypersensitivity
    Chapter 89
    DOG: 1 mg/kg IM once

Tetanus antitoxin (equine)

Tetanus treatment
    Chapters 111, 126, 133
    DOG: Give 0.2 ml SC as a test dose, watch for anaphylaxis
        × 30 min; then give 30,000–100,000 U (100–1000
        U/kg) IM/IV/SC once

Tetracycline HCl (Achromycin V, Panmycin)

Acute tracheobronchitis
    Chapter 16
    DOG: 15–20 mg/kg PO TID
    CAT: 10 mg/kg PO TID
GI bacterial overgrowth, stomatitis
    Chapters 27, 32
    DOG: 10–22 mg/kg PO BID–TID
Brucellosis, chronic leptospirosis, borreliosis
    Chapters 47, 60, 78
    DOG: 10–20 mg/kg PO TID × 28 days
Rickettsial diseases
    Chapters 63, 66, 100, 113
    DOG: 20–22 mg/kg PO TID × 14–21 days
    CAT: 15 mg/kg PO TID × 21 days

Metatarsal fistulation, sterile pyogranulomas, immune skin diseases
   Chapters 82, 85, 89
   DOG: 250–500 mg PO BID, with niacinamide
Episcleritis
   Chapter 96
   DOG: 250–500 mg PO TID, with niacinamide

Tetramisole
Oslerus infestation
   DOG: 2 mg/kg SC × 2–4 Rx

Theophylline (Theolair, Aerolate)
Bronchodilator
   Chapters 12, 16, 17, 18, 132
   DOG: 1–2 mg/kg IV or 5 mg/kg PO TID–QID
   CAT: 1–2 mg/kg IV or 4 mg/kg PO TID
      Sustained release form:
      DOG: 10–20 mg/kg PO BID
      Theodur:
      DOG: 10–20 mg/kg PO BID
      CAT: 25 mg/kg PO SID at night
      Slo-bid:
      DOG: 25 mg/kg PO BID
      CAT: 25 mg/kg PO SID at night

Thiabendazole (Mintezol)
Nasal aspergillosis
   Chapter 14
   DOG: 10 mg/kg PO BID
***Oslerus* infestation**
   Chapter 16
   DOG: 70 mg/kg PO BID × 2 days, then 35 mg/kg PO BID × 20 days

---

Thiacetarsamide (Caparsolate)
Heartworm adulticide
   Chapter 12
   DOG: 2.2 mg/kg IV BID × 2 days

■Thiamine (vitamin B₁)
Seizures
> Chapter 22
> 25–50 mg IM

Thiamine deficiency, malabsorption
> Chapters 32, 120
> **DOG:** 10 mg/kg SC/IM SID × 3–4 days
> **CAT:** 25–50 mg/cat IM/SC SID until signs abate,
> then 10 mg PO SID × 21 days

Ethylene glycol toxicosis
> Chapters 122, 127
> 10–100 mg/kg PO

■Thiamylal sodium (Surital, BioTal)
Anesthesia
> 8–20 mg/kg IV to effect

■Thymosin fraction 5
Growth hormone deficiency
> Chapter 73
> **DOG:** 1 mg/kg SC SID × 7 days

■L-Thyroxine, T₄ (Soloxine, Synthroid)
Hypothyroidism, feline symmetrical alopecia
> Chapters 40, 41, 60, 88
> **DOG:** 22 µg/kg or 0.5 mg/m² PO BID
> **CAT: a)** 20–30 µg/kg/day PO SID or dd BID
> **b)** 0.05–1 mg SID

Myxedema coma
> Chapter 41
> **DOG:** 5 µg/kg IV BID

■Ticarcillin/clavulanate (Timentin)
Septicemia
> Chapter 32
> **DOG:** 40–50 mg/kg IV TID–QID

■Tiletamine/zolazepam (Telazol)
Short-duration anesthesia
> **DOG:** 6–13 mg/kg IM
> **CAT:** 9–12 mg/kg IM

■Timolol maleate 0.25%, 0.5% (Timoptic)
Nonselective β-blocker for glaucoma
> Chapter 98
> Apply 1 drop to affected eye BID

■Tinidazole
Giardiasis
> **DOG:** 44 mg/kg PO SID × 3 days

■Tissue plasminogen activator, alteplase (Activase)
Anterior chamber fibrinolytic
> Chapter 97
> 0.1 ml of 250-μg/ml solution intracamerally

■Tobramycin (Nebcin)
Resistant *Pseudomonas* infections
> **DOG:** 1 mg/kg SC/IM/IV TID

■Tocopherol
> *See* Vitamin A

■Tretinoin (Retin-A)
Canine and feline acne, nasal hyperkeratosis
> Chapter 88
> Apply topically SID–QOD

■Triamcinolone (Vetalog)
Feline plasmacytic pharyngitis, pododermatitis
> Chapter 89
> **CAT:** 2–4 mg PO SID–QOD or 0.4–0.6 mg/kg PO SID, then taper

Triamcinolone (Vetalog) *(continued)*
Anti-inflammatory effects
 DOG: 0.05 mg/kg PO BID–TID
Pemphigus complex
 Chapter 89
 CAT: 0.4–0.8 mg/kg/day PO

Triamcinolone suspension (Kenalog)
Mast cell tumor
 Chapter 91
 2–4 mg intralesionally
Pannus, eosinophilic keratitis, episcleritis, uveitis
 Chapters 96, 97
 DOG: 4–8 mg subconjunctivally
 CAT: 4 mg subconjunctivally

Trientine (Syprine)
Copper hepatopathy
 Chapter 34
 DOG: 10–15 mg/kg PO SID–BID

Trifluridine 1% ophthalmic solution (Viroptic)
Ocular herpesvirus infection
 Chapters 94, 96
 Apply topically 4–8 times daily

Triiodothyronine, T_3 (Cytobin)
Feline symmetrical alopecia
 Chapter 83
 CAT: 20 μg PO BID

Trimeprazine (Temaril)
Antihistamine, allergic skin disease, urticaria
 Chapter 89
 DOG: 0.5–2 mg/kg PO BID

Trimethoprim/sulfadiazine (Tribrissen)
Routine infections
 Chapters 18, 32, 100
 15 mg/kg PO/SC BID

Meningitis
Chapter 24
15–20 mg/kg PO/IM BID
Prostatitis, urethritis, URI
Chapters 51, 52, 112
15–30 mg/kg PO BID
Protozoal polyradiculoneuritis
Chapter 25
30 mg/kg PO BID with pyrimethamine
Toxoplasmosis, coccidiosis, nocardiosis, neosporosis, hepatozoonosis
Chapters 80, 111, 114
15–30 mg/kg PO/SC BID
Bacterial folliculitis
Chapters 84, 85
15–30 mg/kg PO BID
Pneumocystis carinii, **coccidiosis, cyclosporiasis**
Chapter 114
DOG: 15 mg/kg PO BID

Tylosin (Tylan)
GI bacterial overgrowth, chronic colitis
Chapters 32, 33
DOG: 10–40 mg/kg PO BID in food
CAT: 5–10 mg/kg PO BID in food
Feline URI
CAT: 25 mg PO TID
Cryptosporidiosis
Chapter 114
11 mg/kg PO BID × 28 days

Ursodeoxycholate (Actigall)
Chronic hepatitis
Chapter 34
10–15 mg/kg PO SID

Vanadium
Diabetes mellitus
Chapter 43
CAT: 45 mg PO SID, with insulin

Vancomycin (Vancocin)
GI tract bacterial overgrowth
DOG: 3 mg/kg PO BID–TID

Vasopressin
See Lysine-8 vasopressin, Desmopressin acetate, or
Pitressin tannate

Vecuronium bromide (Norcuron)
Paralytic agent for controlled anesthesia
DOG: 10–20 µg/kg IV
CAT: 20–40 µg/kg IV

Verapamil HCl (Calan, Isoptin)
Supraventricular arrhythmias
Chapter 7
DOG: 0.05 mg/kg IV bolus over 5 min, repeat q 10–30 min
to max dose of 0.2 mg/kg

Vidarabine ophthalmic ointment (Vira-A)
Ocular herpesvirus infection
Chapter 94
Apply ⅛ in. topically 5–8 times daily

Vinblastine (Velban)
Mast cell tumor, lymphosarcoma
Chapter 70
1–2 mg/m² IV once weekly, in a protocol

Vincristine (Oncovin)
Transmissible venereal tumor
Chapters 57, 58, 70, 91
DOG: 0.025 mg/kg or 0.5–0.7 mg/m² IV once weekly ×
4–6 wk
Lymphosarcoma, mastocythemia
Chapters 64, 67, 70
DOG: 0.5–0.75 mg/m² IV once weekly, in a protocol
CAT: a) 0.75 mg/m² IV once weekly, in a protocol
b) 0.025 mg/kg IV once weekly, in a protocol

Immune thrombocytopenia
> Chapter 66
> **DOG:** 0.02 mg/kg IV or 0.25–0.3 mg/m^2 IV

Vitamin A (Aquasol A)
Dietary supplement
> Chapters 32, 35
> **DOG:** 100–500 IU PO/IM SID × 10–30 days
> **CAT:** 30–100 IU PO SID

Vitamin A–responsive dermatosis
> Chapter 90
> **DOG:** 10,000 IU PO SID indefinitely

Vitamin B$_1$
> *See* Thiamine

Vitamin B$_{12}$ (Cyanocobalamin)
Dietary supplement
> **DOG:** 100–200 µg/day PO/SC
> **CAT:** 50–100 µg/day PO/SC

Inherited vitamin B$_{12}$ malabsorption, EPI
> Chapters 32, 35, 63, 64
> **DOG:** a) 0.25–1 mg SC/IM weekly for 1 mo, then q 3 mo
> b) 0.5–1 mg IM SID × 7 days, then q 3–6 mo
> **CAT:** 0.1–0.2 mg SC weekly for 1 mo

Vitamin C
> *See* Ascorbic acid

Vitamin D$_2$, ergocalciferol (Calciferol)
Hypocalcemia
> Chapter 42
> 1000–2000 U/kg PO SID, taper to once weekly

Vitamin E (E-Gems, Pure-E)
Scotty cramps
> Chapter 23
> **DOG:** 125 IU/kg/day PO

Vitamin E (E-Gems, Pure-E) *(continued)*
Degenerative myelopathy
  Chapter 24
  DOG: 2000 IU/day PO with aminocaproic acid
Vitamin E–deficient myositis, dermatomyositis
  Chapters 80, 82
  DOG: 200–400 IU PO SID–BID
Acanthosis nigricans, metatarsal fistulation
  Chapter 82
  DOG: 200 IU PO BID indefinitely
Discoid lupus, panniculitis, other immune skin diseases
  Chapters 85, 89
  DOG: 200–800 IU PO, topically BID
Pansteatitis
  Chapter 120
  CAT: 10–20 IU/kg PO BID

Vitamin K₁ (AquaMEPHYTON, Mephyton)
Hepatic cirrhosis
  Chapter 34
  CAT: 0.5 mg/kg SC BID
Warfarin toxicosis, vitamin K deficiency
  Chapters 32, 35, 66, 120, 122, 123
  DOG: 0.5–1.5 mg/kg SC/PO BID–TID × 7–14 days, then
      1 mg/kg/day PO × 4–6 wk
  CAT: a) 5 mg PO SID or 10 mg PO twice weekly
      b) 5–20 mg SC BID for coagulopathy

Warfarin (Coumadin)
Prevent thromboembolism
  Chapters 10, 18, 47
  DOG: 0.1 mg/kg PO SID
  CAT: 0.1–0.2 mg/kg PO SID
  Maintain prothrombin time 2–2.5 times normal

Xylazine (Rompun)
Sedation, muscle relaxant for certain toxicoses
  Chapter 124
  1.1 mg/kg IM/IV

Emetic
> Chapter 122
> **CAT:** 1.1 mg/kg IM

Yohimbine (Yobine)
Amitraz toxicity
> Chapter 87
> **DOG:** 0.1 mg/kg IV

Reverse effects of xylazine and certain toxicoses
> Chapters 122, 124
> 0.1–0.2 mg/kg IV

Zinc acetate
Copper hepatotoxicosis
> Chapter 34
> **DOG:** 50–200 mg PO SID

Zinc methionine
Zinc deficiency
> Chapters 90, 120
> **DOG:** 2–3 mg/kg elemental zinc PO SID

Zinc sulfate (Zinc-220, Vi-Zac)
Zinc deficiency
> Chapters 90, 120
> **DOG:** 2–3 mg/kg elemental zinc PO SID; crush and mix
> with food

Zonisamide (Zonegran)
Seizures
> Chapter 22
> **DOG:** 2–4 mg/kg PO BID

Alphabetical List of Drugs by Brand Name

In the following list of drugs, the generic name is in parentheses.

Acarexx (ivermectin otic solution)
Accutane (isotretinoin)
Acepromazine (acetylpromazine)
Achromycin (tetracycline)
Actidose-Aqua (charcoal, activated)
Actidose with Sorbitol (sorbitol)
Actifed (pseudoephedrine)
Actigall (ursodeoxycholate)
Activase (tissue plasminogen activator)
Adderall (amphetamine SO$_4$)
Adequan (polysulfated glycosaminoglycans)
Adrenalin (epinephrine)
Adriamycin (doxorubicin)
Advantage (imidacloprid)
Aerolate (theophylline)
AErrane (isoflurane)
Alarmucil (psyllium)
Albon (sulfadimethoxine)
Aldactazide (hydrochlorothiazide–spironolactone)
Aldactone (spironolactone)
Alferon (human recombinant interferon)
Alizine (aglepristone)

Alkeran (melphalan)
ALternaGEL (aluminum hydroxide)
Amicar (aminocaproic acid)
Amiglyde-V (amikacin)
Amikin (amikacin)
Aminophyllin (aminophylline)
Amitriptyline (amitriptyline)
Amoxidrops/tabs (amoxicillin)
Amphojel (aluminum hydroxide)
Anadrol-50 (oxymetholone)
Anafranil (clomipramine)
Ancef (cefazolin sodium)
Ancobon (flucytosine)
Android (methyltestosterone)
Android F (fluoxymesterone)
Anipryl (L-deprenyl)
Antilirium (physostigmine)
Antirobe (clindamycin)
Antizol-Vet (4-methylpyrazole)
Apresoline (hydralazine)
AquaMEPHYTON (phytonadione, vitamin K$_1$)
Aquasol A (vitamin A)
Aredia (pamidronate)
Arquel (meclofenamic acid)
Aspirin (acetylsalicylic acid)
Atabrine (quinacrine)
Atarax (hydroxyzine)

Avelcet (amphotericin, liposomal)
Avlosulfon (dapsone)
Axid (nizatidine)
Azium (dexamethasone)
Azopt (brinzolamide 1%)
Azulfidine (sulfasalazine)
Bactocill (oxacillin)
Bactrim (trimethoprim–sulfamethoxazole)
Bactrovet (sulfadimethoxine)
BAL in oil (dimercaprol)
Banamine (flunixin meglumine)
Baytril (enrofloxacin)
Benadryl (diphenhydramine)
Bentyl (dicyclomine)
Berenil (diminazene aceturate)
Betagen (levobunolol 0.5%)
Betapace (sotalol)
Betoptic (betaxolol 0.5%)
Biaxin (clarithromycin)
BioTal (thiamylal sodium)
Blenoxane (bleomycin)
Bonine (meclizine)
Brethine (terbutaline)
Bretylium (bretylium)
Brevibloc (esmolol)
Bromocriptine (bromocriptine mesylate)
Buprenex (buprenorphine)
BuSpar (buspirone)
Butazolidin (phenylbutazone)
Calan (verapamil)
Calcet (calcium carbonate, gluconate)
Calciferol (vitamin D_2)
Calcimar (calcitonin)
Calphosan (calcium lactate)
Caparsolate (thiacetarsamide)
Capoten (captopril)
Capstar (nitenpyran)
Carafate (sucralfate)
Cardioquin (quinidine polygalacturonate)

Cardizem (diltiazem)
CeeNu (lomustine)
Cefa Tabs (cefadroxil)
Celestone (betamethasone)
Cestex (epsiprantel)
Chemet (succimer)
Cheque (mibolerone)
Chloromycetin (chloramphenicol)
Chlor-Trimeton (chlorpheniramine)
Cholac (lactulose)
Cipro (ciprofloxacin)
Citrolith (potassium citrate)
Claforan (cefotaxime)
Clavamox (amoxicillin–clavulanic acid)
Cleocin (clindamycin)
Clomid (clomiphene citrate)
Colace (dioctyl sulfosuccinate)
ColBenemid (colchicine)
Colchicine (colchicine)
Compazine (prochlorperazine)
Conofite (miconazole)
Corid (amprolium)
Cortone acetate (cortisone acetate)
Cosmegen (actinomycin D)
Coumadin (warfarin)
Cuprimine (D-penicillamine)
Cyanocobalamin (vitamin B_{12})
Cystorelin (gonadotropin-releasing hormone)
Cytobin (triiodothyronine, T_3)
Cytosar (cytosine arabinoside)
Cytotec (misoprostol)
Cytoxan (cyclophosphamide)
Danocrine (danazol)
Dantrium (dantrolene)
Daranide (dichlorphenamide)
Daraprim (pyrimethamine)
DDAVP (desmopressin acetate)
Deca-Durabolin (nandrolone decanoate)

Decholin (dehydrocholic acid)
Declomycin (demeclocycline)
Deltasone (prednisone)
Delvosteron (proligestone)
Demerol (meperidine)
Denosyl (SAMe)
Depo-Medrol
    (methylprednisolone
    acetate)
Depo-Provera
    (medroxyprogesterone
    acetate)
Derm Cap (essential fatty
    acids)
DES (diethylstilbestrol)
Desferal (deferoxamine)
Dexate (dexamethasone
    NaPO$_4$)
DHT Tabs (dihydrotachysterol)
Diabinese (chlorpropamide)
Diamox (acetazolamide)
Diapid (lysine-8 vasopressin)
Dibenzyline
    (phenoxybenzamine)
Didronel (etidronate
    disodium)
Diflucan (fluconazole)
Digibind (digoxin immune Fab)
Dilantin (phenytoin)
Dilaudid (hydromorphone)
Diprivan (propofol)
Dithizone
    (diphenylthiocarbazone)
Ditropan (oxybutynin)
Diuril (chlorothiazide)
DMSO (dimethyl sulfoxide,
    40%)
Dobutrex (dobutamine)
DOCP (desoxycorticosterone
    pivalate)
Docusate (dioctyl
    sulfosuccinate)
Donnatal (phenobarbital)
Dopram (doxapram)

Doryx (doxycycline)
Dostinex (cabergoline)
Dramamine (dimenhydrinate)
Droncit (praziquantel)
Drontal Plus (praziquantel)
DTIC–Dome (dacarbazine)
Dulcolax (bisacodyl)
Duragesic (fentanyl
    transdermal patch)
Duramorph (morphine)
Duricef (cefadroxil)
Econopred (prednisolone
    acetate 1%)
Edecrin (ethacrynate sodium)
EFAVet-20 (essential fatty acids)
Efudex (5-fluorouracil)
E-Gems (vitamin E)
Elavil (amitriptyline)
Elspar (asparaginase)
E-Mycin (erythromycin)
Enacard (enalapril)
Enlon (edrophonium chloride)
Enulose (lactulose)
Epogen (erythropoietin)
Eserine (physostigmine 0.25%)
Eskalith (lithium carbonate)
Estratest (methyltestosterone)
Etogesic (etodolac)
Felbatol (felbamate)
Feldene (piroxicam)
Fentanyl citrate injection
    (fentanyl)
Feosol Plus (folic acid)
Fiberall (psyllium)
Filaramide (thiacetarsamide)
Filaribits (diethylcarbamazine)
Flagyl (metronidazole)
Florinef (fludrocortisone)
Fluothane (halothane)
Follutein (human chorionic
    gonadotropin)
Forane (isoflurane)
Frontline Plus (fipronil–
    methoprene)

FSH-p (follicle-stimulating hormone)
Fulvicin (griseofulvin)
Fungizone (amphotericin B)
Furoxone (furazolidone)
Galastop (cabergoline)
Gentocin (gentamicin)
Geocolate (glyceryl guaiacolate)
Glauber's salts (sodium sulfate)
Glucagon (glucagon)
Glucotrol (glipizide)
Glutofac (niacinamide)
GoLYTELY (sodium sulfate)
Grisactin (griseofulvin)
Halotestin (fluoxymesterone)
Heartgard-Plus (ivermectin)
Heparin (heparin)
Herplex (idoxuridine)
Hespan (hetastarch)
Humatin (paromomycin)
Hycodan (hydrocodone bitartrate)
Hydrea (hydroxyurea)
HydroDiuril (hydrochlorothiazide)
Hydromorphone (hydromorphone)
Iberet (ferrous sulfate–folic acid)
Ifex (ifosfamide)
Ilotycin (erythromycin)
Imizol (imidocarb dipropionate)
Immiticide (melarsomine)
Imodium (loperamide)
Imuran (azathioprine)
Inderal (propranolol)
Indorex (pyriproxifen)
INFeD injection (iron dextran)
Inotropin (dopamine)
Interceptor (milbemycin oxime)

Intron (human recombinant interferon)
Isoptin (verapamil)
Isordil (isosorbide dinitrate)
Isovue-200 (iopamidol)
Isuprel (isoproterenol)
Iveegam (human gamma globulin)
Kaopectate (kaolin/pectin)
Keflex (cephalexin)
Kefzol (cefazolin sodium)
Kenalog (triamcinolone)
Ketaject (ketamine)
K-Phos (sodium phosphate)
Lampit (nifurtimox)
Lamprene (clofazimine)
Lanoxin (digoxin)
Lasix (furosemide)
Leukeran (chlorambucil)
Levothroid (levothyroxine, T_4)
Levsin (hyoscyamine)
Librax (chlordiazepoxide–clidinium)
Lidocaine (lidocaine)
Lincocin (lincomycin)
Lioresal (baclofen)
Lithobid (lithium carbonate)
Lithostat (acetohydroxamic acid)
Lomotil (diphenoxylate w/ atropine)
Lotensin (benazepril)
Lotrimin (clotrimazole)
Lutalyse (prostaglandin $F_{2\alpha}$)
LymDip (lime sulfur)
Lysodren (o,p-DDD)
Macrodex (dextran 70)
MCT Oil (medium-chain triglycerides)
Mefoxin (cefoxitin sodium)
Megace (megestrol acetate)
Mephyton (vitamin K_1)
Mestinon (pyridostigmine bromide)

Metamucil (psyllium)
Methotrexate (methotrexate)
Methylprednisolone
(methylprednisolone)
Mexitil (mexiletine)
Milk of Magnesia
(magnesium hydroxide)
Minipress (prazosin)
Minocin (minocycline)
Mintezol (thiabendazole)
Mitaban (amitraz)
Mithracin (mithramycin)
Mitotane (*o,p*-DDD)
Monistat IV (miconazole)
Mucomyst (acetylcysteine)
Mudrane GG (ephedrine)
Muro 128 (sodium
chloride 5%)
Myambutol (ethambutol)
Mycelex (clotrimazole)
Mycolog (nystatin)
Mylanta Calci-tabs (calcium
carbonate)
Myleran (busulfan)
Narcan (naloxone)
Naxcel (ceftiofur)
Nebcin (tobramycin)
Nembutal (pentobarbital)
Nemex (pyrantel pamoate)
Neoral (cyclosporine)
Neo-Synephrine
(phenylephrine)
Neptazane (methazolamide)
Neupogen (granulocyte
colony-stimulating factor)
Neurontin (gabapentin)
Niacin (nicotinamide)
Nilstat (nystatin)
Nipride (nitroprusside)
Nitro-Bid (nitroglycerin 2%
ointment)
Nitrol (nitroglycerin 2%
ointment)
Nitropress (nitroprusside)

Nizoral (ketoconazole)
Nolvadex (tamoxifen)
Norcuron (vecuronium
bromide)
Norpace (disopyramide PO_4)
Norvasc (amlodipine)
Novahistine
(chlorpheniramine)
Novantrone (mitoxantrone)
Numorphan (oxymorphone)
Ocufen (flurbiprofen 0.03%)
Ocupress (carteolol 1%)
Omnipaque (iohexol)
Omnipen (ampicillin)
Oncovin (vincristine)
Optimmune (cyclosporine
0.2%)
OptiPranolol (metipranolol
0.3%)
Orthocide (captan powder,
50%)
Ovaban (megestrol acetate)
Oxyglo$_2$bin (oxyglobin)
2PAM (pralidoxime chloride)
Panacur (fenbendazole)
Pancreazyme (pancreatic
enzymes)
Panmycin (tetracycline)
Paraplatin (carboplatin)
Pavulon (pancuronium
bromide)
Paxil (paroxetine)
Pentam (pentamidine
isethionate)
Pentostam (antimony,
sodium stibogluconate)
Pentothal (sodium
thiopental)
Pepcid (famotidine)
Pepto-Bismol (bismuth)
Percorten pivalate
(desoxycorticosterone
pivalate)
Periactin (cyproheptadine)

Phenergan (promethazine)
Phenobarbital injection
  (phenobarbital)
Pimaricin (natamycin 5%)
Pitocin (oxytocin)
Pitressin (vasopressin)
Platinol (cisplatin)
PMS (follicle-stimulating
  hormone)
Polycillin (ampicillin)
Polyflex (ampicillin)
Portagen (medium-chain
  triglycerides)
Precose (acarbose)
Prilosec (omeprazole)
Primaquine (primaquine PO_4)
Primaxin (imipenem)
Primor (sulfadimethoxine/
  ormetoprim)
Principen (ampicillin)
Prinivil (lisinopril)
Procan SR (procainamide)
Profasi (human chorionic
  gonadotropin)
Profenal (suprofen 1%)
Profigil (modafinil)
Proglycem (diazoxide)
Program (lufenuron)
ProHeart-6 (moxidectin)
Pronestyl (procainamide)
Propantheline (propantheline)
Propecia (finasteride)
Prostaphilin (oxacillin)
Prostigmin (neostigmine)
Protamine (protamine)
Protopam (pralidoxime)
Protropin (growth hormone)
Proventil (albuterol)
Provera (medroxyprogesterone
  acetate)
Prozac (fluoxetine)
Prussian blue (ferric
  cyanoferrate)
Pure-E (vitamin E)

Purinethol (6-mercaptopurine)
Quadrinal (theophylline–
  ephedrine)
Questran (cholestyramine)
Quinidex (quinidine SO_4)
Quinidine (quinidine SO_4)
Rapinovet (propofol)
Reglan (metoclopramide)
Regumate (altrenagest)
Requa (charcoal, activated)
Retin-A (tretinoin)
Revolution (selamectin)
Rheomacrodex (dextran 40)
Ridaura (auranofin)
Rifadin (rifampin)
Rifamate (rifampin)
Rimadyl (carprofen)
Ripercol (levamisole)
Ritalin (methylphenidate)
Robaxin (methocarbamol)
Robinul (glycopyrrolate)
Rocaltrol (vitamin D_3)
Roferon-A (interferon)
Rompun (xylazine)
Salix (furosemide)
Sandimmune (cyclosporine)
Sandostatin (octreotide
  acetate)
Seldane (terfenadine)
Serax (oxazepam)
Serophene (clomiphene
  citrate)
Sinequan (doxepin)
Slo-bid (theophylline)
Solganal (aurothioglucose)
Soloxine (levothyroxine)
Solu-Cortef (hydrocortisone
  sodium succinate)
Solu-Delta-Cortef
  (prednisolone sodium
  succinate)
Solu-Medrol
  (methylprednisolone sodium
  succinate)

Somophyllin (aminophylline)
Soriatane (acitretin)
Sporanox (itraconazole)
SSKI Solution (potassium iodide)
Stilphostrol (diethylstilbestrol)
Streptomycin (streptomycin)
Strongid-T (pyrantel pamoate)
Sudafed (pseudoephedrine)
Sulfadiazine (sulfadiazine)
Sulfodip (lime sulfur suspension)
Surfak (dioctyl sulfosuccinate)
Surital (thiamylal sodium)
Synthroid (levothyroxine, T_4)
Syntocinon (oxytocin)
Syprine (tetramine)
Tagamet (cimetidine)
Tapazole (methimazole)
Tardak (delmadinone acetate)
Tavist (clemastine)
Telazol (tiletamine/zolazepam)
Temaril (trimeprazine)
Tenormin (atenolol)
Tensilon (edrophonium chloride)
Terramycin (oxytetracycline)
Theo-Dur (theophylline)
Theolair (theophylline)
Thiola (2-mercaptopropionyl glycine)
Thorazine (chlorpromazine)
Timentin (ticarcillin–clavulanate)
Timoptic (timolol maleate 0.5%)
Tofranil (imipramine)
Torbugesic (butorphanol tartrate)
Torbutrol (butorphanol tartrate)
Tracrium (atracurium besylate)

Tramisol (levamisole)
Tranxene-SD (chlorazepate dipotassium)
Trental (pentoxifylline)
Trexan (naltrexone)
Tribrissen (trimethoprim/sulfadiazine)
Trusopt (dorzolamide, 2%)
Tumil-K (potassium gluconate)
Tums (calcium carbonate)
Twin-K (potassium gluconate)
Tylan (tylosin)
Tyson (L-carnitine)
Urecholine (bethanechol)
Urobiotic-250 (oxytetracycline)
Valium (diazepam)
Vancocin (vancomycin)
Vasotec (enalapril)
Vasoxyl (methoxamine)
Veetids (penicillin V)
Velban (vinblastine)
Ventolin (albuterol)
Versed (midazolam)
Versenate (calcium EDTA)
Vetalog (triamcinolone)
Vibramycin (doxycycline)
Viokase (pancreatic enzymes)
Vira-A (vidarabine)
Virilon (testosterone cypionate)
Viroptic (trifluridine 1%)
Vitamin C (ascorbic acid)
Vi-Zac (zinc sulfate)
Voltaren (diclofenac 0.1%)
Winstrol (stanozolol)
Wycillin (procaine penicillin)
Xalatan (latanoprost 0.005%)

Xanax (alprazolam)
Yobine (yohimbine)
Zantac (ranitidine)
Zinc-220 (zinc sulfate)
Zithromax (azithromycin)

Zofran ODT (ondansetron)
Zoloft (sertraline)
Zonegran (zonisamide)
Zyloprim (allopurinol)

Classification of Drugs by Generic Name

ANTIBIOTICS/ ANTIBACTERIALS

Amikacin
Amoxicillin
Amoxicillin–clavulanic acid
Ampicillin
Azithromycin
Cefadroxil
Cefazolin sodium
Cefotaxime
Cefoxitin sodium
Ceftiofur
Cephalexin
Chloramphenicol
Ciprofloxacin
Clarithromycin
Clindamycin
Clofazimine
Cloxacillin
Doxycycline
Enrofloxacin
Erythromycin
Ethambutol
Gentamicin
Imipenen
Isoniazid
Lincomycin
Metronidazole
Minocycline
Ormetoprim–sulfa
Oxacillin

Oxytetracycline
Paromomycin
Penicillin, aqueous
Penicillin, procaine
Rifampin
Streptomycin
Sulfadiazine
Sulfadimethoxine
Sulfadimethoxine–
   ormetoprim
Tetracycline
Ticarcillin–clavulanate
Tobramycin
Trimethoprim–sulfadiazine
Tylosin
Vancomycin

ANTIDOTES/THERAPIES FOR TOXINS

Acetylcysteine
Acetylpromazine
Amphetamine SO_4
Apomorphine
Ascorbic acid
Atipamezole
Atropine SO_4
Calcium EDTA
Charcoal, activated
Deferoxamine
Digoxin immune Fab
Dimercaprol (BAL)

Diphenhydramine
Diphenylthiocarbazone
Ethanol 20%
Ferric cyanoferrate
Glyceryl guaiacolate
Glyceryl monoacetate
Hydrogen peroxide
Ipecac
Lime water
Magnesium hydroxide
Methocarbamol
4-Methylpyrazole
Nicotinamide
D-Penicillamine
Physostigmine
Potassium permanganate
Pralidoxime chloride
Protamine sulfate
Pyridoxine
Sodium bicarbonate
Sodium sulfate
Sodium thiosulfate 20%
Succimer
Tetanus antitoxin
Thiamine
Xylazine
Yohimbine

ANTIFUNGAL AGENTS

Amphotericin B
Captan powder 50%
Clotrimazole
Enilconazole
Fluconazole
Flucytosine
Griseofulvin
Itraconazole
Ketoconazole
Miconazole
Natamycin
Nystatin
Potassium iodide
Rifampin

Sodium iodide
Thiabendazole

ANTI-INFLAMMATORY DRUGS

Acetylsalicylic acid
Betamethasone
Carprofen
Chlorpheniramine
Clemastine
Colchicine
Cortisone acetate
Cyproheptadine
Dexamethasone
Diphenhydramine
Etodolac
Flunixin meglumine
Hydrocortisone sodium
 succinate
Hydroxyzine
Meclofenamic acid
Methylprednisolone
Methylprednisolone acetate
Methylprednisolone sodium
 succinate
Niacinamide
Phenylbutazone
Piroxicam
Polysulfated glycosaminoglycans
Prednisolone
Prednisolone sodium
 phosphate
Prednisolone sodium
 succinate
Promethazine
Terfenadine
Triamcinolone
Trimeprazine

ANTIPARASITIC/ ANTIPROTOZOAL DRUGS

Albendazole
Amitraz

Amprolium
Benzimidazole
Clindamycin
Diethylcarbamazine
Diminazene aceturate
Epsiprantel
Fenbendazole
Fipronil
Furazolidone
Imidacloprid
Imidocarb dipropionate
Ipronidazole
Ivermectin
Levamisole
Lime sulfur suspension
Lufenuron
Meglumine antimonate
Melarsomine
Methoprene
Metronidazole
Milbemycin oxime
Moxidectin
Nifurtimox
Nitenpyran
Paromomycin
Pentamidine isethionate
Praziquantel
Primaquine PO_4
Pyrantel pamoate
Pyrimethamine
Pyriproxifen
Quinacrine
Selamectin
Sodium stibogluconate
Sulfadiazine
Sulfadimethoxine
Tetramisole
Thiabendazole
Thiacetarsamide
Tinidazole

BEHAVIOR MODIFIERS

Alprazolam
Amitriptyline

Buspirone
Chlorazepate dipotassium
Clomipramine
Diazepam
Fluoxetine
Hydrocodone bitartrate
Medroxyprogesterone acetate
Methylphenidate
Naloxone
Naltrexone
Paroxetine
Sertraline

CARDIOVASCULAR DRUGS

Acetylpromazine
Amlodipine
Atenolol
Atropine SO_4
Benazepril
Bretylium
Calcium chloride
Calcium gluconate
Captopril
Chlorothiazide
Digoxin
Diltiazem
Dobutamine
Dopamine
Enalapril
Epinephrine
Ethacrynate sodium
Furosemide
Glycopyrrolate
Heparin
Hydralazine
Hydrochlorothiazide
Isoproterenol
Isosorbide dinitrate
Lidocaine
Lisinopril
Methoxamine
Mexiletine
Morphine SO_4
Nitroglycerin 2%

Nitroprusside
Phenoxybenzamine
Phenylephrine
Phenytoin
Prazosin
Procainamide
Propantheline
Propranolol
Quinidine
Sodium bicarbonate
Sotalol
Spironolactone
Taurine
Terbutaline
Verapamil
Warfarin

DERMATOLOGIC DRUGS

Acitretin
Amitraz
Amitriptyline
Auranofin
Aurothioglucose
Calcitriol
Captan powder 50%
Chlorpheniramine
Clemastine
Clofazimine
Clomipramine
Clotrimazole
Dapsone
Diphenhydramine
Doxepin
Essential fatty acids
Fluoxetine
Fluoxymesterone
Griseofulvin
Hydroxyzine
Imipramine
Isotretinoin
Melatonin
Methylprednisolone acetate
Miconazole

Naltrexone
Niacinamide
Nystatin
Pentoxifylline
Phenobarbital
Potassium iodide
Prednisolone
Promethazine
Sodium iodide
Terfenadine
Tretinoin
Trimeprazine
Vitamin A
Vitamin E

**ENDOCRINE/REPRODUCTIVE
DRUGS**

Acarbose
Aglepristone
Altrenagest
Antidiuretic hormone
Bromocriptine
Cabergoline
Calcitonin
Calcitriol
Calcium gluconate
Chlorothiazide
Chlorpropamide
Chorionic gonadotropin
  (human)
Clomiphene citrate
Cortisone acetate
Danazol
Delmadinone acetate
Demeclocycline
L-Deprenyl
Desmopressin acetate
Desoxycorticosterone pivalate
Dexamethasone
Diazoxide
Diethylstilbestrol
Erythropoietin
Etidronate

Finasteride
Fludrocortisone
Fluoxymesterone
Follicle-stimulating hormone
Gallium nitrate
Glipizide
Glucagon
Gonadotropin-releasing
  hormone
Growth hormone
Hydrochlorothiazide
Insulin, NPH
Insulin, PZI
Insulin, regular
Insulin, ultralente
Ketoconazole
Liothyronine (T_3)
Lysine-8 vasopressin
Megestrol acetate
Methimazole
Methylprednisolone acetate
Methyltestosterone
Mibolerone
Mithramycin
Mitotane
Octreotide acetate
Oxytocin
Pamidronate
Pitressin tannate
Prednisolone
Progesterone
Proligestone
Prostaglandin $F_{2\alpha}$
Pseudoephedrine
Spironolactone
Stanozolol
Stilbestrol
Tamoxifen
Testosterone cypionate
Testosterone, methyl
Testosterone proprionate
Thymosin fraction 5
L-Thyroxine (T_4)

Triiodothyronine (T_3)
Vanadium

GASTROINTESTINAL DRUGS

Ascorbic acid
Atropine SO_4
Bisacodyl
Bismuth
Chlordiazepoxide–
  clidinium
Chlorpromazine
Cholestyramine
Cimetidine
Cisapride
Clidinium
Colchicine
Dehydrocholic acid
Diazepam
Dimenhydrinate
Dioctyl sulfosuccinate
Diphenoxylate
Famotidine
Flunixin meglumine
Glycopyrrolate
Hyoscyamine
Kaolin/pectin
Lactulose
Lomotil
Loperamide
Magnesium hydroxide
Meclizine
Medium-chain triglycerides
Methylprednisolone
Metoclopramide
Metronidazole
Misoprostol
Nizatidine
Omeprazole
Ondansetron
Oxazepam
Pancreatic enzymes
D-Penicillamine
Prednisolone

Prochlorperazine
Propantheline
Psyllium
Ranitidine
SAMe
Sucralfate
Sulfasalazine
Triamcinolone
Trientine
Ursodeoxycholate
Zinc acetate

IMMUNOSUPPRESSIVE/ CYTOTOXIC/ CHEMOTHERAPEUTIC AGENTS

Aclarubicin
Actinomycin D
Asparaginase
Auranofin
Aurothioglucose
Azathioprine
Bleomycin
Busulfan
Carboplatin
Chlorambucil
Cisplatin
Cyclophosphamide
Cyclosporine
Cytosine arabinoside
Dacarbazine
Dexamethasone
Doxorubicin
5-Fluorouracil
Hydroxyurea
Ifosfamide
Lomustine
Melphalan
6-Mercaptopurine
Methotrexate
Methylprednisolone acetate
Mitoxantrone
Piroxicam

Prednisolone
Triamcinolone
Vinblastine
Vincristine

NEUROLOGIC DRUGS

Acetazolamide
Bethanechol
Clorazepate
L-Deprenyl
Dexamethasone
Diazepam
Dimethyl sulfoxide, 40%
Edrophonium chloride
Felbamate
Gabapentin
Imipramine
Iohexol
Iopamidol
Mannitol
Methocarbamol
Methylphenidate
Methylprednisolone sodium succinate
Modafinil
Neostigmine
Pentobarbital
Phenobarbital
Potassium bromide
Prednisolone
Pyridostigmine bromide
Yohimbine
Zonisamide

OCULAR DRUGS

Acetazolamide
Betamethasone
Betaxolol 0.5%
Brinzolamide 1%
Carteolol 1%
Cyclosporine 0.2–2%
Dichlorphenamide
Diclofenac 0.1%

Disodium EDTA 1%
Dorzolamide 2%
Flunixin meglumine
Flurbiprofen 0.03%
Glucose 40%
Glycerin
Idoxuridine 0.1%
Latanoprost 0.005%
Levobunolol 0.5%
Mannitol
Methazolamide
Methylprednisolone acetate
Metipranolol 0.3%
Miconazole
Natamycin 5%
Physostigmine 0.25%
Pilocarpine 1%
Prednisolone
Sodium chloride 5%
Suprofen 1%
Taurine
Timolol maleate 0.5%
Triamcinolone
Trifluridine 1%
Vidarabine 3%

RESPIRATORY DRUGS

Albuterol
Aminophylline
Butorphanol tartrate
Chlorpheniramine
Dexamethasone
Doxapram
Ephedrine
Epinephrine
Furosemide
Hydrochlorothiazide
Hydrocodone bitartrate
Hydrocortisone sodium
  succinate
Isoproterenol
Prednisolone
Prednisolone sodium
  succinate

Pseudoephedrine
Terbutaline
Theophylline

TOPICAL/CUTANEOUS MEDICATIONS

Amitraz
Captan powder 50%
Chlorhexidine 0.5%
Clotrimazole
Lime sulfur suspension
Nystatin

TRANQUILIZERS/ ANESTHETICS/ ANALGESICS

Acetylpromazine
Buprenorphine
Butorphanol tartrate
Chlorpromazine
Diazepam
Fentanyl
Halothane
Hydromorphone
Isoflurane
Ketamine
Meclofenamic acid
Meperidine
Methocarbamol
Midazolam
Morphine
Oxymorphone
Pentobarbital
Phenobarbital
Propofol
Sodium thiopental
Thiamylal sodium
Tiletamine/zolazepam
Xylazine

Narcotic Antagonists:
Naloxone
Naltrexone

Paralytic Agents:
Atracurium besylate
Pancuronium bromide
Vecuronium bromide

URINARY TRACT DRUGS

Acetohydroxamic acid
Allopurinol
Aluminum hydroxide
Ammonium chloride
Ascorbic acid
Baclofen
Bethanechol
Calcitriol
Chlorothiazide
Cisapride
Dantrolene
Diazepam
Dicyclomine
Diethylstilbestrol
Dobutamine
Dopamine
Ephedrine
Erythropoietin
Ethacrynate sodium
Furosemide
Imipramine
Mannitol
Megestrol acetate
2-Mercaptopropionyl
   glycine
Nandrolone decanoate
Oxybutynin
D-Penicillamine
Phenoxybenzamine
Phenylpropanolamine
Potassium citrate
Prednisolone
Propantheline
Sodium bicarbonate
Stanozolol

VITAMINS/MINERALS/ SUPPLEMENTS

Ascorbic acid (vitamin C)
Calcitriol
Calcium carbonate
Calcium gluconate
Calcium lactate
L-Carnitine
Dihydrotachysterol
1,25-Dihydroxyvitamin D_3
Ergocalciferol (vitamin D_2)
Essential fatty acids
Ferrous sulfate
Folic acid
Iron dextran
L-Lysine
Magnesium sulfate
Medium-chain triglycerides
Pancreatic enzymes
Phytomenadione (vitamin K_1)
Potassium chloride
Potassium gluconate
Potassium phosphate
Safflower oil
Sodium bicarbonate
Sodium chloride
Sodium phosphate
Taurine
Thiamine (vitamin B_1)
Vanadium
Vitamin A (tocopherol)
Vitamin B_{12}
   (cyanocobalamin)
Vitamin E
Zinc methionine
Zinc sulfate

MISCELLANEOUS DRUGS

Aminocaproic acid
Coumarin
Cyproheptadine

Danazol
Desmopressin
Dextran 40 or 70
Dextrose 50%
Diosmin
Gamma globulin, human
Granulocyte colony-
    stimulating factor
Heparin
Hydroxyethyl starch
Hypertonic saline 7.5%
Interferon
Lithium carbonate
Mithramycin

Nandrolone decanoate
Oxazepam
Oxyglobin
Oxymetholone
Pamidronate
Polysulfated
    glycosaminoglycans
Rutin
Sodium bicarbonate
Sodium chloride
Sodium phosphate
Stanozolol
Tissue plasminogen activator
Yohimbine

NOTES

NOTES

NOTES

NOTES

NOTES

NOTES

NOTES